The
Strength
of Love

Kate Garraway

The Strength of Love

Embracing an Uncertain Future with
Resilience and Optimism

BLINK
bringing you closer

First published in the UK by Blink Publishing
An imprint of The Zaffre Publishing Group
A Bonnier Books UK company
4th Floor, Victoria House
Bloomsbury Square,
London, WC1B 4DA
England

Owned by Bonnier Books
Sveavägen 56, Stockholm, Sweden

Hardback – 978-1-788707-40-4
Trade Paperback – 978-1-788707-41-1
Ebook – 978-1-788707-42-8
Audio – 978-1-788707-43-5

A CIP catalogue of this book is available from the British Library.

Designed by Envy Design Ltd
Printed and bound by Clays Ltd, Elcograf S.p.A

1 3 5 7 9 10 8 6 4 2

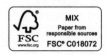

Blink Publishing is an imprint of Bonnier Books UK
www.bonnierbooks.co.uk

This book is dedicated to all those facing a fearful and unpredictable tomorrow... let love, in its myriad forms, be our beacon.

Contents

Hello Again!

I'm so pleased to at last bring you my book. I was supposed to have written it at the beginning of 2022. That was the plan but, as the old saying goes, life got in the way.

When I last put pen to paper to you in 2021 to write *The Power of Hope*, Covid was the only story in town. We were gripped by fear, trapped in our homes and separated from our loved ones. Hugging anyone outside our 'bubble' was illegal and it felt as though surviving the pandemic was the greatest challenge we'd ever have to face.

My husband Derek had caught Covid in March 2020 and, when that book was published, he was still in hospital, unable to speak or move. We prayed that one day he would come home to us – and many of you were kind enough to send us messages of support, willing us to keep fighting on, just as you were fighting on too. Without it ever being our intention, it felt as though Derek's fight for life and our family's struggles had somehow come to represent the fears and struggles that everyone was enduring at that time: to keep themselves and their loved ones safe from this deadly virus.

After more than a year of Derek's life hanging in the balance, our prayers were finally answered and we were told he could come home. At the same time, it seemed that the world's prayers were being answered too, with the development of effective Covid vaccines and treatments prompting a relaxation of restrictions. We all dared to believe that the worst might be over and that maybe we could return to the lives we had known before, wiser and more appreciative of the things we'd been missing, determined to make every second count.

It hasn't quite worked out like that for our family; and I wonder whether, whatever your circumstances, you feel it hasn't quite worked out that way for you either.

While mercifully the pandemic seems to have been consigned to history, you might be finding that you're still worried about the future and that everything feels more precarious maybe even than before. We are, after all, in the middle of one of the worst economic crises in living memory, with no clear end in sight.

While some emerged from lockdown with renewed spirit, inspired to pursue different career directions or to improve their work-life balance, the reality is that many businesses built on decades of hard work have gone under and many others are struggling to stay afloat. Thousands of people are scrabbling to find enough money to cover essentials, such as food, heat and shelter. Hundreds of thousands are grieving and millions more are suffering from long Covid, the effects of which are still not fully understood. On top of that, other health worries have been exacerbated by long waiting lists and huge treatment backlogs and we are starting to question whether our beloved NHS is strong enough to cope.

The mental health epidemic, which was bubbling under the surface before Covid, seems to have erupted just when resources are stretched to breaking point. Marriages and relationships are under strain, and some question whether the struggle is worth it, wondering is *this* what we stayed in our homes for, worked long hours for, made sacrifices for? The collective mood is low and it feels as if genuine happiness is in short supply.

I know I am lucky in so many ways and I can never fully express my gratitude to the doctors, nurses and health workers who have got us this far. But nevertheless, the happy ending I desperately wanted to bring you still eludes us. I really wanted to give you a story of how love conquers all, to deliver the uplifting end to our grim family saga that your loyalty and support deserves. I hoped to be able to tell you that Derek is stronger and happier – that he is better – and that our family is feeling renewed, energised and living every day to the full, our collective trauma fading into distant memory.

I would love to be able to tell you that since Derek has been home everything has been easy, that the miracle of having him with us has turned the day-to-day challenges into a breeze. But the truth is that the fear of him dying has never left us, because he's been rushed back to hospital so many times, and every time we live with the fear that *this* crisis will be the one that takes him from us.

There have been times when I've wondered whether, if I couldn't deliver a triumphant story of Derek's recovery, I had anything to offer in a book at all. I wanted to give you something you might read and use to face whatever challenges you have in your own life. I wanted our story to inspire you to think 'If they can get through that, so can I.' How wonderful it would have been to be able to deliver all the answers wrapped up in a neat bow.

But that's not real life, is it? There are no easy solutions, no smug happy endings, no clear conclusions because life will always throw you a curveball just when you least expect it. Sometimes the curveballs are big, sometimes they're smaller, but whichever they are, they keep coming and the trick is learning how to deal with them. That is what this book will give you. In sharing some of the things I have learned to help me stay strong and resilient, I hope it helps you too.

Not that there haven't been plenty of golden moments in our long dark tunnel. I have experienced the joy of

Hello Again!

Derek's incredible spirit and I remain blown away by him and his ability to power on. If I'm honest, though, there have been times when the stress of fighting for safe care at home, and support to help ease Derek's symptoms, has threatened to do what Covid never did: break my resilience. I will share some of these darker moments with you in this book.

The good news is that it never did quite break me, though; and I wouldn't have been able to finish this book if I hadn't felt I could share enough hope to help you find a way through your own hard times.

My struggle is still very much a work in progress, and I will share in these pages everything that's helped me through so far and the practices that are setting me on a happier path. One of the most important things I have learned is to recognise and appreciate the power of love in all its forms. The love of friends is as irreplaceable and as valuable as any I have experienced, as is the love between a child and their parent or carer, or between siblings, or wider family. There is love in the jokes shared with colleagues and love in the kind words shared by a stranger. And when you are on the receiving end of love and kindness from others, it fuels you to get through the next minute, hour or day. There is power in giving love too – whether it be someone you adore or a stranger you meet in passing.

Love is everywhere if we choose to look for it ... and research tells us it is exactly what we need to help us cope with pain: a hug when we're suffering might not make everything better, but it certainly helps. Scientists have discovered that painkillers target the same areas in the brain that are activated by intense love – and you don't even have to be touching or talking for these effects to be felt. Just the presence of someone you love can make you more resilient to pain.

Neuroscientists now believe that if one of the cerebral areas involved in love gets damaged through illness or injury, the brain seeks other neural pathways to make love happen. In other words, if one of the brain systems, circuits or transmitters that powers love fails, there's a back-up. Our brain won't let love go. It's like having a generator in your shed in case of a power outage – but it's a generator that can take over from your main power supply permanently, if need be. And that's why love is such a strong energy in the world, such a mighty force of nature. The brain is constantly finding new ways of keeping love alive.

Love is the force that drives us to look for the connection we need, as human beings – and that sense of connection creates so much good in the world and also helps us to deal with the bad. It's what links us in a society and bonds us across oceans. Perhaps all those songwriters are right – love really does make the world go round.

The fact is, our brains are wired for love: when we feel loved, the neural pathways connected with negative emotions like fear and embarrassment are altered, freeing us to kiss a lover in the street or strip off on a summer night and splash around in a river; and love is associated with the regions of the brain that relate to empathy, tolerance, emotional stability, and a more positive outlook. When we feel this way, our bodies are at their healthiest and the evidence shows that those in long-term happy relationships generally have longer, healthier lives.

But just as love can make us, it can also break us. Heartbreak is a killer, an actual condition with a medical name, *takotsubo syndrome* or *stress cardiomyopathy*, and it can be caused not just by the ending of romantic love but by other types of loss and grief.

Getting the love I need, from those around me, is what sustains me every day – and you are all part of that, along with my wonderful family, friends and colleagues.

There was a point on this journey, though, when it felt as if the weight of love was about to break me – and that, I think, is where our story together should start …

Chapter 1

The Crash

November 2022. I woke with a start as my alarm sounded. It was 2am and time to get up and go and present *Good Morning Britain*. My bed was as warm as a giant hug, and I did *not* want to leave it. Mind you, this was nothing new. Anyone who works shifts knows that the law of the alarm clock always dictates that you are in your deepest, most restful sleep of the night at the exact moment it goes off. Even if you haven't slept a wink before, you will always be deep in slumber when that annoying sound starts.

'Urgh, nothing for it,' I thought. 'I've got to get up, out of this cosy cocoon.' I tried to reach for the off-button before the alarm woke everyone else in the house.

But my arm wouldn't move.

I tried again, this time attempting to turn towards the alarm clock, but again nothing happened. Without moving my head, I cast my eyes down my body, feeling I needed to check it was still there. My hands were on top of the duvet, tightly clenched and pointing upwards at a strange angle, like I was ready to sling a right hook. 'Put 'em up,' I thought to myself, recalling the Cowardly Lion in *The Wizard of Oz* and I wanted to laugh out loud at the thought but no sound came out. I must have looked so ridiculous.

I tried to relax and uncurl my fists but couldn't. It was like having an out-of-body experience; except I hadn't escaped my body – my body seemed to have escaped me. For a second I wondered if I was actually still asleep, having one of those dreams when it feels as if you are trying to run but you're unable to move your legs.

The alarm was still blasting away.

'Mum, for God's sake, what's going on? Turn that thing off!' Darcey screamed from the room next door. 'Just get up and go to work, or you'll be late!' she added.

Nope, I was definitely awake.

'Right,' I thought, 'I can do this. It must just be stress or something; I need to relax.'

I took a deep breath in, and breathed out very slowly. Then I did it again, this time trying to make a big 'aahh' sound as I breathed out. This is a technique my friend Gouri, a Reiki practitioner, taught me. Focusing on making the sound stops you thinking about anything else; the vibration of the vocal cords stimulates your vagus nerve, which is part of your parasympathetic 'rest and digest' nervous system; the vagal response regulates your internal organ functions and helps you relax by calming your heart rate and blood pressure.

For so many years, religions and new age practices have involved some form of singing or humming. While in a religious setting, we sing for the communal spirit and to give praise which is uplifting in itself but it also works on a physical level to benefit us too. Activating our vocal chords in any setting – even in the shower or a karaoke booth! – releases huge amounts of tension in the body and stimulates endorphins. It's funny how so much knowledge has been lost or forgotten and now has to be ratified scientifically before we will accept it again.

I breathed in deeply and, focusing only on my breath, almost shouted a huge *aaahh!!!*

'Wow, that was loud!' I thought. 'At least I can speak – that's one ability I definitely need to do the show!'

Now to get out of bed. 'Don't think about it,' I told myself. 'Just do it. There's definitely something weird going on, but don't focus on that, focus on the normal – do what you always do.'

I was talking to myself the way I had heard therapists in hospital speak to Derek when they were trying to encourage him to move. Covid had damaged the neural connections between his brain and his limbs, and it was as if he had forgotten how to lift his hand; they tried distracting him, so he would move instinctively, on automatic pilot, using muscle memory.

I took another deep breath and let out the biggest *aaahhhhh* I could. It was *so* loud.

'Quiet!' shouted Darcey from next door, in exactly the same tone Derek used to use when I was driving him mad, teasing him about something or other. It made me giggle and, distracted by the laughter, I rolled out of bed onto my knees.

'Phew,' I said, then almost immediately, 'Aarrrrrgggh!'

There was a searing pain in my chest – as though someone had punched their fist through my breastbone, snatched hold of my heart and squeezed. The pain was sharp and excruciating.

Then I realised that it wasn't a sudden onset of pain. It had actually been there all the time – not as fierce maybe, but definitely there. My brain just hadn't been feeling it somehow. My temporary paralysis had distracted me from it, or maybe adrenaline had prevented me from feeling it. Whatever this pain was, I was now *very* aware of it, and I panicked. 'Don't!' I told myself. 'If it *is* your heart, panicking will make it worse.' Then came the thought, 'Oh God, was I having a heart attack?'

Still on my knees, I threw up onto a pile of papers next to my bed.

I hauled myself up to go to the bathroom, panting, and stubbed my toe on a box file. 'Damn it! I should have moved that!' I thought, then remembered why I had left it there: it was full of reports and forms to be filled in later that day, for Derek's hospital appointments. I had hoped that leaving it in the middle of the floor would remind me to fill them in. I thought of all the things I had to do that day, on top of *GMB* and my Smooth Radio show.

I was startled by a banging on the front door. I looked at the clock – it was 2:40. It must be the driver wondering where the heck I was ... I was already late.

'Coming!' I shouted, trying to sound convincing.

'Right,' I said to myself, 'come on, Garraway, take it one step at a time. Don't think about anything apart from getting in the shower and then into the car. This is what you are good at: getting on with it; tackling the biggest priority in front of you, not getting swamped in what might or might not happen. Just focus.'

I stumbled out of the bedroom, across the landing, into the bathroom and promptly threw up a second time. I had to acknowledge that the pain was really bad now. I sat, focused on my breathing and then got into the shower.

The shower helped a bit. Just enough for me to get downstairs and open the front door, where a panicked driver was waiting on the doorstep, fretting about how late we were.

'Are you okay? I was worried.'

'Just one of those mornings, you know,' I said, trying to hide the fact that I wasn't at all sure what kind of morning this actually was.

The Strength of Love

People have been so kind to me and my family ever since Derek got sick. Maybe it's because he got sick just as the world feared it might get sick too. When the early reports about Covid started coming through, none of us seriously believed it would affect us. Then, as the nation was gripped by it and Derek caught it and fought it, everyone saw him as an example, either of what they feared might happen to them or of what *had* happened to them.

Not a day goes by when people don't stop to ask how Derek is and how the children are, to ask me to send their love to both. Others share their experiences of caring for their loved ones. 'Keep going, it's worth it,' they say.

It's wonderful to receive so much love. But I also sense a longing. I see a look in their eyes, one that says they really want me to tell them everything is okay, that the battle has been won, that their prayers have been answered, that Derek is fighting fit again, being the dad he wants to be and the husband he would love to be. I desperately want to give them that happy ending – almost as desperately as I want it for myself.

It's such a privilege to see people at their best, showing the type of kindness that life's trials can sometimes obscure. Some days there will be a post on Instagram from someone who relates; or another person might squeeze my shoulder when I'm on the Tube. 'Keep going, you can do it.' But then I see a shadow, an ache from the challenges of their own life, that makes me wish more than ever that I could tell them all has turned out well and *they* will get there too.

The driver had that look in his eye. He had his own troubles, no doubt. He didn't need mine on top of his.

I gave him a smile in the rearview mirror.

'LBC news is on the radio – I tuned in because I know you like it. And the light is on in the back for reading. All good to go?' he said.

'Perfect. Yes, let's do this.' I managed a big smile and a positive nod for emphasis.

Opening my folder, I started looking at the briefs the *GMB* researchers had sent – the notes on the guests we will be interviewing. Of course, we make sure we are up to date on the news anyway, but these briefs have details of anything new that has broken overnight. I usually love reading them – it's as if you are jumping into the show from the moment you open your folder in the morning taxi. The day has begun and you can get swept up in it – framing questions you want to ask, thinking of things you might do or say, and the pictures that could be used. I always scribble down the questions I want to ask the producers, or details I'd like to follow up. It's exciting and I can't wait to get in and get on. But this particular morning I somehow couldn't engage; nothing I was reading seemed to stick. The words didn't so much swim on the page as sit there frozen.

I started to feel slightly dizzy, so I opened the car

window. It was one of those mild November mornings that we often have in London, when the air is warm and thick with fine, misty rain – not driving and freezing rain, like we get in February but more blankety and soft.

It was still long before dawn; and as the car whizzed through the dark, the speed whipped the fine rain into my face. It felt good. When I'm out of sorts, especially emotionally, immersing myself in the natural world always helps. Whether it be getting my hands dirty in the soil when gardening, lying on the grass and feeling it tickle my skin while I gaze up at the unfathomable expanse of the sky, getting soaked in the rain or frozen in the snow, or being battered by waves in the sea. Sometimes when I am lost in fear in my head or consumed by analysing my problems, just connecting with the outside world can be healing. That connection overrules my thoughts for a moment. It takes me out of my head and into something bigger than myself. It somehow reconnects brain and body, allowing feelings to flow yet still be contained. It makes me feel part of something huge, rather than an isolated fragment; it reminds me of the scale of the world around me, like a big pinch that wakes me up and puts my troubles into context.

Maybe it was the grounding feeling that came with this blast of nature that meant I could allow thoughts of what had happened only an hour earlier to seep back into my mind. I sat there with my shower-wet hair, letting the rain soak my face, and suddenly it wasn't rainwater on my cheeks – it was tears. Floods of sobless tears streaming down my face. It was as though my feelings had found a way to escape a tank that I'd tried to seal.

I thought of how I'd felt when I'd woken up – the awful sensation of being trapped, paralysed. I knew that must be how Derek feels every morning, when he wakes up and can't move. He's not in control of his body or mind, imprisoned – except, for him, there is no chance of breaking free, no getting up and getting on. He is caught in the state Covid has left him in: alive, yes, and so grateful for that, but still not living a life with purpose, not even close. He is unable to really express love, to be a part of the lives of those he loves in any meaningful way, unable to do his psychology work (his passion); unable to party with his friends or to indulge in the hobbies that used to inspire him. The things he loved are all still there; he is still there but trapped – unable to connect. The damage, his injuries, mean they are always just out of reach – and we are unable to reach him too.

But why was *my* body reacting like this? Could I be so desperate to help Derek that I'd started having sympathy pains? Was I also trapped by his sickness, by his incapacity? Or was I actually sick too? (Oh God, who would look after our poor kids?) Or had I been fighting for so long that my body was preparing for battle – fists up, rigid against the onslaught – even while I slept?

Why was I still in crisis? Shouldn't I have moved

on by now? How had I failed to take control? Was I as okay as I assured everyone I was? It seemed I was still in the adrenaline-fuelled fighting state I was in on the day Derek went into hospital. The war to keep him alive was far from won, so the battle had to carry on, didn't it? The fight to save him and our family, the fight that friends had praised me for undertaking: was this fight actually damaging *me*? And what did that mean for the children? I was still in a constant state of fear that I might lose him because his situation was still so precarious. Only weeks earlier, Derek had been blue-lighted back into hospital with another life-threatening development. Again, I'd had the fear of losing him; the crisis just went on and on.

The pain in my chest was back. It had never really gone away, just been pushed aside, smothered by my need to get on with things. But now it was overwhelming, and I couldn't ignore it.

We were coming off the dual carriageway, nearing the *GMB* studios, when nausea swept over me. There was no doubt – I wasn't going to make the last half mile to the loo in the dressing room.

'Excuse me, do you think you might be able to pull over for a moment?' I asked the driver, trying to sound casual and breezy.

'Are you okay? Am I going the wrong way? What's wrong?'

Clearly, I hadn't managed to pull off 'breezy'.

'It's okay, I just need a bit of air. Sorry, I didn't mean to worry you!'

We pulled over. I jumped behind some recycling bins and was sick in the kerbside drain.

'God, how shameful! I hope no one saw,' I thought. At this hour of the morning, I probably looked like a drunken partygoer spilling her guts at the end of a night out. I cringed at the thought of mums and kids passing this spot on their way to school a few hours later.

I went back to the car. 'Do you have any water?' I asked the driver, hoping he thought I just wanted a drink.

'Sure, loads: grab a bottle from inside the door.'

I scuttled back and flushed the sick away down the drain as best I could, hoping that the residents of this quiet suburb would never know what had happened.

'Ow!' I yelped, as I got back in the car.

'Careful,' said the driver, maybe thinking I'd bashed my knee as I climbed in.

But it was the pain in my chest, which was now all-consuming and creeping up my neck and into my jaw.

I didn't attempt to read any more and closed my eyes instead, not because I wanted to sleep (there was no chance of that) but to try and steady myself ... It helped a bit but didn't touch the pain. Then the car turned into the *GMB* car park and pulled up outside the entrance to the dressing rooms.

Pre-Covid, I would always have gone straight upstairs

to the production office when I arrived, got a brew on the go, logged on to the computer and gone through the running order with the producers. When the Covid restrictions hit, we were confined to our dressing rooms and briefings were done first on the phone, and then in small groups. Everyone got used to being segregated so we'd have laptops in our dressing rooms and prepared alone. At 5am the editor, as now, gave a joint briefing with the presenters, before going on air.

I really missed the 'old way'; I used to love walking into a busy newsroom where teams of journalists had been working all night. The camaraderie offset the brutality of those early starts.

If most people turned up at their workplace at 3am, it would be eerily deserted; they would have to flick the lights on and try to shake themselves into action. But at 3am, *GMB*'s newsroom is buzzing. Reports are being edited, headlines rewritten, graphics designed to illustrate complicated issues, and there is a sense that the countdown to the big on-air moment is underway. You feel as if you are meant to be awake, that you are where the action is, at the centre of a busy, spinning world. It feels like high noon, not the middle of the night.

This particular morning, though, I was relieved not to have to go to the newsroom or see anyone. I thanked the security guard who had opened the dressing-room door for me and, without even switching on the light, slumped on the sofa.

This was not good. The pain was not going away – a giant sharp lump stuck in my chest, spreading up to my collarbone on the left side, through my neck and into my jaw.

Had I pulled something? Could this be a muscular strain?

I tried to think of what I had been doing over the previous couple of days.

No new exercises, certainly – it's been years since I've had a chance to go to the gym. Even digging and weeding my beloved garden, which is my escape and always rejuvenates me, has been sadly neglected, with plants waiting to be potted and bulbs not yet planted for next spring. I certainly couldn't blame the pain on that.

Of course, there was caring for Derek at home. He wasn't the chubby, cuddly pre-Covid Derek, who I could never have attempted to lift – Covid had wiped eight stone off him in a matter of weeks. But, despite that, at six foot two, he was still way too heavy for me to heave, even in his weakened state. This is because, without the ability to move, he is a dead weight; you don't realise just how much difference tensing muscles makes until you try to lift someone who can't. He needs constant repositioning in bed; we have to pull him up and on to a kind of manual hoist so we can get him out of bed for a full wash and to change his sheets. And we are still having challenges getting the right care for him at home; it is a constant battle with the care system, not least because Derek's care is so novel; it doesn't fit into any pre-existing assessment process.

The battle is exhausting and demoralising, but the chance to care for Derek is so uplifting. I want to do it, it makes me feel closer to him and it was what I prayed to be able to do during those endless terrible days when him being home seemed too much to hope for, when his life could have been snatched away at any second. I have always been careful to follow the guidance about how to move him, to protect my back as well as his, but even with Darcey and Billy's help, it was still a struggle, and I was finding it harder and harder as time went on. Maybe I, too, was being weakened; maybe firing on all cylinders for such a long time had used up every last drop of fuel in my reserve tank.

Had I worn myself out and broken my body through the act of caring? Had love broken me?

'Surely not,' I told myself. 'You are being melo-dramatic!' After all, I had been caring for Derek since he came out of hospital in April 2021, so why would I be in this pain now?

The battle had gone on for so, so long. I couldn't think of it as temporary any more. It wasn't a case of 'getting through it' and then being able to relax. With each step forward we seemed to take two more back.

The battle to get support and care at home was not going away, either. I had already completed reams of appeals documentation, which so far amounted to six box files of reports, attempting to prove to the authorities that Derek was so damaged that he warranted care at home, even though anyone who saw him for a few seconds knew instantly that he needed that support. There had also been many meetings that took days to prepare for. Because Covid was such a new disease, very few medical scientists realised just how much damage it could cause, and those who did were specialists on extreme hospital wards, not in the community.

When Derek was first released from hospital, we were assured he would get 24-hour care to meet his primary healthcare needs. But it wasn't made clear how long for and in fact it was only for a matter of weeks. In the meantime, I'd been running up terrifying amounts of debt to keep Derek safe and at home.

'Stop this!' I shouted out loud, conscious that I was spiralling downwards. 'Get a grip and get on with the job; don't start thinking about all these problems. Get on with the show.'

I turned on the light. Ooh, mistake – too bright. I flicked the light on in the adjacent bathroom instead and left the door ajar so there was just enough light to see by.

'Okay, think clearly: it's now nearly four o'clock and the pain isn't going away. If I don't let someone know my predicament now, it's going to cause a massive problem... What the heck will they do about the show? Who will host it?'

Don't get me wrong, I knew I wasn't indispensable. This is something that all presenters know – at any point any one of us could be replaced by someone newer, younger or simply better. It's not that TV bosses are cruel or that the industry is more brutal than any other; far from it, in my experience. Yet I have always been very aware that it isn't a job for life. Maybe no job is. When I first started on ITV Breakfast Television 23 years ago, my old boss, Peter McHugh (now sadly passed away), said, 'No one has the deeds for the "sofa"; we are all just tenants, so always remember you are lucky to be here. Many came before you and many will come after you. Have as much fun as possible, work as hard as you can to get as good as you can and look after your life outside of work, as you will need it.'

He looked grey and sad as he added, 'Don't make work your life, because it could be taken away at any point, not through any fault of your own. That is just the nature of telly, and maybe the nature of life itself.'

I don't know if he gave this speech to every newbie who joined the sparkly, exciting world of *GMTV*. Perhaps he had forgotten that I'd already spent several years in TV, at ITV regions, the BBC and SKY, and knew the 'all that glisters isn't gold'. Or maybe he knew that being on *GMTV* was different from those other shows.

Breakfast television presenters have a unique emotional connection with viewers, which is something I've always really treasured. When you watch TV in the morning, you're often at your most wobbly and vulnerable – you've just staggered out of bed and you're probably pouring yourself a cup of coffee. When viewers see us in person and come up and say hi, they often tell us: 'I'm usually in my pants and pyjamas when I'm watching you!'

I think that creates a wonderful bond. It means that people feel a connection to you – and you feel connected to them. It's not quite the same as sitting down with your tea on a Saturday night to watch a big entertainment show, which is more like going to the theatre. In the morning, it's as if the presenters have popped round to your house and you feel you know them well enough to invite them in, even in your pyjamas. It's a different connection. We are not 'stars', we're more like mates. Unlike newsreaders on evening news bulletins, we have always shared our lives with the people who watch, and they share theirs with us, so it all has a bit of a 'one big family' feel. But we still have to be very professional.

It's work and you have a responsibility to your colleagues and to the viewers to get it right. So you take the job seriously but, in my view, not yourself or your position. Yes, there's the excitement when you go on air, the adrenaline rush from making sure you get a breaking news story right. The fun and banter you have with your co-presenters and the extraordinary and famous people you have the privilege of interviewing – it's all thrilling. But just as the red light goes on, it also goes off; you need a *real* life too.

Ironically, though, it was my working life that had sustained my home life since Derek had been sick. Everyone at *GMB* and Smooth Radio, from the first moment, had been so supportive: sending me love and food parcels in the days when we were in lockdown and we couldn't visit each other; rearranging work rosters to accommodate every setback and drama that cropped up at short notice. Ranvir Singh and Charlotte Hawkins have both had to scrap many personal plans at the last minute in the last three years to cover for me on air; Tina Hobley and Myleene Klass do the same thing on Smooth; Susanna Reid even came into the studio in the middle of her annual holiday to do the show, just so that the kids and I could spend time with Derek in hospital when we finally got the chance to visit. And Ben Shephard, Richard Arnold and Piers Morgan were always available day and night for pep talks.

Being at work has helped me mentally, too. It gives me the chance, for a few hours, to be the person I had been before Derek became sick and, maybe just as importantly, be reminded of the life I had lived before Derek and I had even met. It reconnected me with my 'old self', so I didn't feel completely submerged by the crisis. Being there – showing up and being professional – was vital for my self-esteem. And of course the reaction from viewers and listeners meant more than I can ever express. In return, I could give a voice to those who were alone and suffering, and speak up for carers, which gave me renewed professional purpose. Getting back to work when Derek was starting to show signs of recovery had normalised things as much as anything could.

I owed my colleagues so much, and the last thing I wanted to do was let them down.

'Right, I need to tell someone … I can't keep hiding in the dressing room – and this pain is not going away.'

I phoned the newsroom and spoke to Jen, the editor overnight and for the show that morning. I didn't really know what I was going to say. It was all going to cause a big problem and I didn't want to be 'the problem' yet again.

'Jen, it's Kate. I hate to cause a panic, but I really don't feel well. I know it sounds dramatic, but I don't feel good at all. I have a terrible pain in my chest. And I just feel grim.'

'I will be right down,' she said.

She was there in minutes. 'Hi!' she said, laughing and smiling. 'What the heck's going on with you?' she teased, as she looked round the door. Then her face fell.

Clearly, I looked ashen and terrible. The fact that I didn't make one of my usual jokes about her seeing me without makeup probably told her even more about how bad I was feeling.

'Oh no, are you okay?'

'Yes, yes, sorry to be a nuisance,' I said. 'It's just that I have this terrible pain in my chest; I've had it since I woke up this morning. I've been sick too: when I woke up and again in the car. I don't think it's gastric.' It didn't feel like a tummy bug.

'Where is the pain?'

'Here.' I pointed to the middle-left area of my chest. 'And it keeps spreading over here, into my arms and up my neck, left side and into my jaw.'

With my finger I traced the flow of pain, like storm fronts on a weather map. Laura Tobin, *GMB*'s meteorologist, would have been proud of me. But I couldn't quite believe I was saying it out loud to someone else; suddenly it was real.

'God, Jen, I am so sorry! This is the last thing you need just before the show,' I continued. 'I don't know what to do. I am sure I will be fine; it's just that the pain isn't going away ... I don't think it's gastric,' I said again. 'I don't know what it is.'

'Right, right, okay,' she said, buying herself time to think, clearly realising it was not okay. 'Don't apologise – we can sort it ...'

'It could be a panic attack maybe, or some kind of extreme indigestion?' I said, trying to think of something that could potentially play itself out before I went on air. Something that could be solved. As I'd never had a proper panic attack, I had no idea what that might feel like. I didn't think I'd eaten anything unusual the day before – but at that point I couldn't remember what I *had* eaten.

'I don't think it's a heart attack – it can't be!'

And there it was, like a rock landing in a pond: the fear that I hadn't wanted to allow into my thoughts all along.

'No, I'm sure it's not,' she said quickly; then, gathering herself, she went on, 'Right, what to do? I am going to call Dr Hilary [breakfast TV's doctor to the nation for over 30 years].'

That's the first thought for anyone who works in ITV breakfast television who has any medical worry – in fact, I had called Dr Hilary on the day Derek first became sick and it was he who had told me to call an ambulance.

'Oh no, don't!' I said. 'I don't want to wake him up in the middle of the night.'

'He won't mind. He's around. Also, I think we may have a doctor in the building – let me try that, too. I am going to sort it out and get someone to sit with you. Stay there.'

In a flurry of what I'm sure was panic, she ran off.

Then the deputy editor appeared. 'Okay, we are on it. I can't get hold of Hilary. I left a message and we don't have a doctor on site. What does it feel like? Should I call an ambulance?'

'No, no, that seems so dramatic, I'm sure it's nothing – maybe try Dr Amir.'

Dr Amir had been really supportive that week, helping me with the reports I had been preparing for Derek's care appeal. For months, he'd been helping me process all the notes I had taken over the past three years or so, supporting me as a kind of clinical advocate while I got back in touch with the many specialists and healthcare professionals who had treated Derek in the nine hospitals he had been admitted to since he first got sick. Only that week, we'd had another crunch meeting, the outcome of which was supposed to be a final decision on how Derek could be kept safely at home. (In the event, the decision was delayed yet again – for how long we didn't know.) So I was confident Amir would understand the bigger picture.

'Maybe text him, so it doesn't wake him up unnecessarily, and then if he's awake he will call back,' I suggested.

But before he was able to ring back, Hilary returned the producer's call. They spoke for a bit, with Alex (the producer) trying to spell out the seriousness of the situation without wanting to worry me even more. We all looked to Hilary for calm reassurance and he knew that I was listening.

I heard him say a long drawn-out, 'Okaaay, let me speak to her ...'

'Hi Hils,' I said. 'So sorry to wake you. It's the last thing you need on the one day you are not getting up to work on *GMB*.'

'Don't worry, it's a GP's life!' His voice is always so reassuring. 'Now, what's going on with you?'

I ran through my symptoms and he asked me questions. Then he asked if, while we had been chatting, I'd still been feeling pain. I said that I had.

'Where?'

'Centre of tummy, centre of chest, up into shoulder, neck and jaw.'

He said another long 'Okaaay' and asked to be passed back to Alex.

Even though she had the phone pressed against her ear, the dressing room was quiet so I could hear everything. Hilary said, trying to sound calm, 'Right, I think we do have to get her to hospital. I'm sure it isn't a heart attack, but it is *Kate* we're talking about. And we know what she's got going on. And we know what she's already been through. She's never talked about anything like this before, so I think we have to take it seriously. Call an ambulance.'

'Okay,' she said.

'Don't do that, Alex,' I interrupted. 'They are so busy, it'll take ages to come. I'll just go to the hospital.'

'I'll deal with it, Hilary. Don't worry,' Alex said, and hung up.

'Don't call an ambulance,' I pleaded. 'Honestly, I'm sure it's nothing and I'll never get back in time to do the show.'

She looked at me in disbelief. 'Kate, there's no question: you're *not* going to do the show. I can't believe you're still thinking that. We've messaged Charlotte. She's going to step in and we're going to get you to hospital. It's probably just stress because of all that you are dealing with, but we have to get it checked out.'

And there it was. The thing that I had perhaps most dreaded hearing. Of course, I was under stress, but I didn't want to give in to *that*; I didn't want to acknowledge it, to let it into my thoughts. It couldn't be a heart attack – I refused to even think that. A heart attack was something that couldn't be powered through, and powering through was my survival tactic. My mantra was: keep going with positivity and eventually everything comes good.

But what if it doesn't? What if the one you love doesn't get better? What if you get sick, too? What if you aren't helping your kids through the biggest trauma of their lives … then what do you have left? Plus, if I couldn't even be a good employee, I felt lost.

I was the one who always kept going at work, who showed up with a smile – even when I was on my knees, for heaven's sake. I had carried on when I was pregnant, throwing up in the bin in the ad breaks; I had struggled in with kidney infections and limped in with broken toes.

In the last two and a half years, I'd pushed on through after being up all night, when Derek's life was hanging in the balance, when I had been talking to him on FaceTime from his intensive-care bed as he spiralled downwards, saying he couldn't go on. I'd told him he *could* go on, reminding him of all he had to live for and telling him that he would love life again; that this was just the beginning, that he was going to get *himself* back and life was going to be better than ever. I told him that he had purpose: that he was still a father, a husband, a son, a brother, a friend; that he was needed and loved in all these roles and he was going to get them back. He wasn't going to get trapped in this purgatory. I'd watched over FaceTime as he'd sobbed – him in his hospital bed, me in our bed at home – seeing the clock tick closer to the time when I had to get up for *GMB*, not having had any sleep.

I had kept on going, even when the children were so frightened that they had gone beyond crying to silent sobs and into quiet sleep, when I had hugged them and stroked their hair in my bed – getting them through it.

Keeping going, being the resilient one, was what I clung on to, as something I could still achieve, something I could still offer to all those who had given me so much. Without that, what use was I to ITV? What was the point of me being on the roster at all?

I was never the most talented presenter, but I *always* delivered. Over the years I had often joked with bosses that I might not be the best, but I was the best they could get for the money. 'At least I am good value,' I'd say, 'and hopefully, even when I do muck up, the joke's on me, so it gives people a laugh!'

To compensate, I would always get in early and do endless prep to prove that I was reliable – but now I was a let down.

'Definitely don't call an ambulance,' I told Alex. 'I'll get a taxi.'

'In that case, we'll have to find someone to go with you,' she said.

From then on, it's all a bit of a blur. They found a junior producer called Charlie to come with me – an adorable young lad in his twenties. I'd only met him a couple of times before and we'd probably said two or three words to one another in a professional capacity, while he handed briefs over to me. Now he appeared at my door not knowing what the hell he was going to find. He found me looking absolutely crazy – my washed hair had dried into a massive frizz-ball, and I was clearly in a lot of pain.

We headed out to the cab. 'Let's go to University College Hospital, it's near and I know they have a big A&E,' I managed to say.

He tried to make conversation but I just felt so faint that I put my head between my knees. Then Dr Amir phoned me back, having got the earlier message. He asked me to go through what was happening and tell him my symptoms. 'Just try and keep calm,' he said, and then he asked to speak to Charlie and also told him to do his best to keep me calm.

'Have you had a nice week?' Charlie asked. 'What have you been up to with the kids?' Bless him. I could tell he felt so responsible. I had to say, 'Charlie, I'm sorry. I don't think I can talk, but I really appreciate you trying!'

When we arrived at the hospital, we almost literally fell into A&E. 'I think I'm going to have to lie down,' I said, and collapsed on the floor. I felt absolutely terrible by this point and A&E was so bright that my eyes couldn't take the light. Even I could no longer deny that this might really be something as devastating as a heart attack.

While I lay like a crazy woman in the middle of the floor, Charlie attempted to get someone's attention. He was trying to tell the person at the triage desk my name, give them some details to go on and, I could tell, was trying to be discreet, thinking that I wouldn't want anyone to recognise me.

'Tell them I'm Kathryn Draper,' I whispered, thinking he might be worried about someone recognising my name. 'I am officially in the system as Mrs Draper.'

They found my file and tried to get me to get up to see a nurse, but I was only half-aware of what was going on. Eventually the triage nurse came over and said, 'How much has she had to drink and has she taken any drugs?'

They were clearly used to dealing with badly inebriated club and partygoers at this hour in the morning.

They couldn't actually see who I was because I was lying in a heap on the floor, my hair covering my face.

'She's not had any drink or drugs,' Charlie said. 'She's just been at work.'

'What does she work as?'

'She works in television, at ITV.'

'Why is she working at this time?'

'It's an early morning show,' he said.

He was really trying to be discreet and avoid saying *Good Morning Britain*, but in fact it just came across as evasive. It was just making them more suspicious that it was drugs or drink, and they thought I was being difficult by not getting up. 'If she doesn't get up, we'll call security. I mean it: get her up and at least onto a chair – she can't just lie there like that.'

Just then, Amir rang again. 'I'm trying to explain, but they seem to think she's drunk or on drugs,' Charlie told him.

'Hang on, Charlie,' I called. 'Help me up and get me into a cubicle, or something.'

Charlie tried, but probably assumed I just needed a bit of a lift, a hand up – not realising the deadweight half-faint I was in. As a result, we lost our balance and fell on each other. Poor Charlie! He struggled to scoop me up, half-carrying, half-dragging me across the room. Eventually he got me into a wheelchair and the staff began to see that this was something different. Suddenly I was swept into a first response area, where they quickly put monitors on my chest, took blood tests and blood pressure rates and measured oxygen levels in my blood.

By now Oruj, *GMB*'s editor of the morning, had arrived at the hospital. She'd managed to get the show on air and had dashed over to support Charlie.

She was relatively new to the job, and it was one of my first shifts with her. She was probably wondering what the hell was going on. I felt I wasn't making a great impression!

'I'm so sorry; I can't believe I've caused all these problems – you really don't need this,' I said. 'You go back, it's fine, they are looking after me now.'

'Don't be silly, I want to be here.'

A cardiologist came and gave me painkillers, which helped, and explained that they were waiting for results and would be back. Oruj started to watch *GMB* on her phone to monitor how it was going. Hearing the show was strangely comforting and I found myself drifting into something resembling sleep.

Eventually the cardiologist came back and wanted to speak to me on my own.

'We have your ECG back,' he said. (An ECG is an electrocardiogram, which records the heart's activity through electrodes placed on the skin.) 'And you'll be pleased to know it shows you are not having a heart attack right now. Unfortunately, that doesn't mean there isn't a problem. Actual attacks are incredibly hard to capture in the moment unless you just happen to be there.'

He then went on to talk about blood test results and heart attack indicators. He told me about something called troponin, which I gathered is a protein that isn't normally found in the blood but is released when the heart is in distress. A heart attack happens when blood flow to the heart is blocked – and high levels of troponin in the blood can be an indicator of a heart attack and other heart problems.

'There are lots of issues with your heart that we still can't rule out,' he added, 'so we definitely need to get to the bottom of it, and we will. How are the pains now?'

'Better,' I said. 'Still there, but not sharp and pressing like before.'

'Well, we can either keep you here for 12 hours, or we can send you home as you live so near. I think you will sleep and rest better at home. We'll bring you back later in the day for more tests. But,' and, he stressed, it was a big but, 'if you feel anything like the sharp pain you had before, you *must* come back straight away. And do *not* go back on air.'

He had been so kind and I felt relieved. I reasoned that they wouldn't let me go if it was *that* serious, would they? So I grabbed the chance to get home. Before I left, he said, 'It's a huge pleasure to meet you. You're such an inspiration and my wife loves you. She's a carer for her mother and we both think you're doing so much good by speaking out on things.'

I started to cry. 'I'm not doing any good for anybody,' I said. 'You're the ones who are doing good; look at you, you're the ones who are here saving people. I'm not doing anything.'

'No, you are doing good. Keep going, it's really important that people like you speak out.'

I thought, 'But I'm literally failing on every front right now: my kids, because I'm not there with them; Derek, because I can't do all I need to do for him; work, because I'm here at the hospital instead of presenting the show … and *you're* thanking me!'

His kindness made me feel so guilty and at the same time amazed at how wonderful people are.

'Look, whatever is going on with the pain in your chest – and we will find out – I think what you have to face, Kate, is that you're under incredible stress, and whatever is happening today is at the very least a warning. It is going to affect you and damage your health, so you have to take care of *you*,' he went on. 'Are you taking time for yourself?'

I wanted to laugh out loud – but I didn't because I knew he meant it in such a caring way. Of course I know that looking after myself is the right thing to do but how do you realistically do that when you are spinning so many plates? If you stop them spinning for even a second, one will crash. It was an unwinnable situation but I knew I had to resolve it. I couldn't carry on living on adrenaline if I was in danger of making myself sick – I'd be leaving the kids without any parent and letting down everybody around me.

He left with a smile, and I told Oruj I could go home. Relief all round and, before I knew it, I was in a cab thinking, 'What the hell happened this morning?' While trying to get to grips with it, I turned to humour, which is what I always do because if I can laugh at a situation, it feels less serious.

I looked at my phone and saw a message from Ben Shephard saying, 'Garraway, what's going on? Heard you have had a drama. Is it a heart attack, or is it wind?' Clearly, he wasn't aware how serious it was and he was just being his usual teasing self! He knew that whatever I was really going through, this would normalise things – it's just the way we are with each other.

I replied with a voice message: 'Don't worry, I'm on my way back. I don't quite know what it is. I'm having more tests later. But I must tell you about this. Poor Charlie, you know, that lovely producer. He had to carry me across A&E – I'm not joking, Ben, it was like a scene from *An Officer and a Gentleman!* Poor, poor guy, and you know how heavy I am! It's probably scarred him for life.'

Immediately a voice note pinged back, with him singing (dreadfully), 'Up Where We Belong' from the movie's soundtrack, and laughing about it helped me feel better, for a moment.

Then I realised I was nearly home. Thank God, the kids had already left for school. Derek's sister, Di, was staying; she had come to help out, as she had done so many times, as all of Derek's family and mine had tried to do. Again, she had rearranged her work, put off important things she had to do in her own life, left her partner behind and come down to be with us. How could I walk into the house, tell her the latest news and give her more worry?

'This has to stop,' I thought. 'I have to get off this tortuous merry-go-round – but how?'

All around me, I could feel love and kindness coming from every direction: the cardiologist saying thank you; Charlie trying to be nice; Oruj coming to support me; Ben texting to see how I was; Charlotte covering for me. All of them reaching out the hand of love. I knew I couldn't ask any more of anyone else, but I also knew I was at crisis point.

I couldn't work any harder or longer. I couldn't make any more money to pay for more care for Derek. I couldn't do any more to help Derek recover. I was chasing every referral going for Derek, but there were so many delays (just as there were for everyone) and the waiting only seemed to lead to more risk for him, more fear, more unknowns and uncertainty. I couldn't be with the kids any more than I was, or any less. I couldn't slice the pie of time any better because there were too many hungry mouths to feed, and I had to find more than crumbs for myself or there wouldn't be any pie left to share. I had to make a change. I just didn't know what it was yet.

Chapter 2

Adrenaline – My Frenemy

There's comfort in knowing that the Earth goes through seismic changes over millennia. The ground erupts, landscapes fold up, mountains crumble, oceans shrink to puddles or subsume great tracts of land – and still life continues. The natural world is in flux, but the life force goes on – creatures adapt to changed habitats and climates. Miraculously, they thrive again.

But, just as certainly, there will always be another earthquake ...

In my world, two and a half years after Derek had become catastrophically ill, the ground beneath my feet was threatening to break up again. My dash to hospital was an early warning on my personal seismometer, telling me that living in long-term readiness for fight or flight was posing a risk to my health, with implications for all those around me. Love might be giving me my best chance of keeping a solid foothold, but fear and uncertainty were undermining its power. I knew I was far from alone in feeling this insecurity, as both of these menaces have been in our lives for so long now.

Can anyone actually remember a time when they didn't feel anxious about the future, unstable in the present and craving the past? (Hasn't the past always, in some ways, seemed like a mythical era when everything was, well, the opposite of scary and uncertain, when life was reliable, and even our worries more manageable?) Now the present felt even more precarious than ever. We were being attacked from all sides. Not just all the usual worries about our elderly relatives, job dissatisfaction, the cost of living, you name it, but Covid, the fallout of financial uncertainty, job insecurity and fear of losing our homes. And post-Covid, we've also been asking ourselves: 'How do I help an anxious child who's finding the school years hard? Christ, while I have been struggling to get online *and* get my kids online, what have they been doing on social media all this time? Have I been too distracted to notice that their sense of identity has lost its footing and is now dangling perilously above a river of likes and dislikes?'

Was there ever a time this hard? How can we get through it? Even people who remember the war, or the Seventies and the three-day week, tell me they feel this is somehow worse because this time there's so much anger in the atmosphere, born of a sense of betrayal, a feeling that we've been let down, of promises – spoken or unspoken – having been broken. Political instability and rising inflation have added to our sense of insecurity. The people and the structures we thought we could rely on to protect us from life's ups and downs no longer feel like they offer the safety net we expect.

There is a sense that the cavalry isn't coming, that we are somehow on our own and don't know where to turn for help. Some frustrations have been simmering for a while, but the infuriating shortcomings of modern life have taken on a new urgency as we face the current cost of living crisis. During the pandemic a sense of community gave us some comfort, yet even that now feels like it's breaking down. We fear that everything that we have worked hard for and take pride in is being stripped away, as we struggle to cut back and work even longer hours, just to provide the basics for our families – like food and heat.

The climate crisis is another huge ever-present problem that seems impossible to solve as an individual and, politically, there is a sense of pointlessness. That somehow life is deeply unfair; that while we patiently wash out jam jars, big corporations and governments around the world are doing nothing; that somehow, in a way that supersedes party politics, the odds are stacked against us.

Meanwhile, those who try to instigate change often

make our lives tougher in the short term. Even if you agree with the cause and the action being taken, life is tough enough to navigate without train drivers and teachers being on strike, or protesters disrupting major events, which you've been looking forward to in order to escape the real world for a moment. Doctors are setting up food banks and health workers are using them. Kids are walking around hungry and malnourished, with holes in their shoes. And who has heard of nurses ever striking before? On top of that, doctors and consultants are too. Not to mention ambulance and bus drivers, train and highway workers, baggage handlers, driving instructors and staff at the Royal Mail and Border Force – all desperate, all saying enough is enough. There is a sense that our world is somehow broken, its spirit crushed.

Maybe ironically, the event that rocked the foundations of my world came at a time when I had never felt more stable. I was back from the jungle after my stint on *I'm a Celebrity*, where I'd bonded with my campmates and surprised myself by getting through some utterly disgusting challenges. I had come out feeling really quite good about myself. Work was going well and there were offers of new jobs in the pipeline. Derek was excited about setting up his new business. The kids were happy and doing well at their new schools. Life felt great.

Derek and I were like honeymooners after I'd been in the jungle, separated from the outside world, for 22 days. I had missed my family so much, and it made me realise all over again how much I loved Derek, how much I depended on him – for support, intimacy, laughter, conversation and so much more. When I stepped off the bridge that led out of our camp and collapsed into his great big loving bear-hug, I was already home. It felt that good, that comforting – and at the same time, the smell and the feel of him made me dizzy with a renewed sense of the strength of our love.

Our first night back together, after so long apart, was unbelievably romantic. We even started planning to renew our wedding vows the following summer. It wasn't going to be a reset – we didn't need that – so much as a reaffirmation of what we already knew; that after 19 years, we were still as much in love as ever. The world felt bright and shiny, as if polished with happiness. The future was ours for the relishing and I was determined to work out, get fit and eat nothing but gorgeous, healthy, kangaroo- and insect-free healthy food. I felt so lucky.

But life can change in a heartbeat; it can change in an hour or a day. And ours did.

I think we all have days in our lives that, even as we are living them, we know we will remember forever. And at any point in the future, a smell or a piece of music can instantly transport us back to that day and the emotions we felt. Romance, joy, exhilaration, triumph – or the less good experiences, like getting into trouble at school, being dumped, or saying goodbye to a loved one forever. We don't necessarily think of these moments every day:

it takes a memory jog, a reminder – sad or happy – to transport you back.

Yet I relive 30th March, 2020, when Derek first went into hospital, when everything changed for our little family. Every day I relive the fear, the guilt, the grief, the hope, the failure and the love – perhaps most of all the love. Painful, excruciating, exhilarating, transforming love. I don't even need a smell, or a tune, to remind me; I live those emotions every minute in brilliant technicolour. It's as if that day still hasn't ended and its consequences go on and on, like a Groundhog Day. Try as you might, you still wake up back there, just like Bill Murray in the movie every time the alarm clock went off. With each new morning you think 'A new chance! I will change the outcome, avoid the traps, learn lessons and make progress,' but somehow there's another twist that puts you right back where you started.

Maybe you too have days in your past that haunt you like this, that imprison you. It's like being trapped, isn't it? Stuck on a rollercoaster that never ends, an adrenaline-induced trance that keeps you upright but one you can never break out of.

Considering that March day triggered the most dramatic change our family could ever have encountered, it actually started breathtakingly normally. My usual 2:15am *GMB* alarm woke me with a start. Every time it shocks me awake, even after 25 years. Derek was sleeping next to me; he had been feeling 'under the weather' for

48

a few days and couldn't seem to shake it off, which was unlike him. We had rung the GP, who asked if he had a cough or a temperature. No, just a blistering headache, dizziness and an indescribable feeling of exhaustion. She didn't ask about loss of smell – no one even knew that was a Covid symptom then – but did ask if his nose felt blocked and whether he'd had sinusitis before.

He said he had, adding that it felt worse than that somehow, but that it might be a bad case of it. He pressed his sinuses on his cheekbones and on his forehead as he thought about it ... yes, they hurt.

To our amazement, she quickly prescribed a course of antibiotics, apparently eager to get him off the phone. Her priority wasn't patients with possible sinusitis – something treatable and curable – it was the increasing number of patients presenting with Covid.

I looked at Derek sleeping seemingly peacefully. 'Good,' I thought, 'hopefully the antibiotics are kicking in.' And then I got in the taxi to go to the *GMB* studio, opened my pack of briefs and started to plough through the big stack of newspapers.

The headlines were all about Covid. Not the daily death figures that dominated our lives for so many months afterwards; this was still the point when only the most vulnerable were thought to be at any real risk; when the debates all seemed to hint at the risk being fairly academic. The comical elbow taps that replaced handshakes seemed rather silly, the subject of comedy.

Even the wearing of masks was still being questioned. One doctor on *GMB* that morning suggested that mask-wearing could potentially increase the likelihood of infection because it encouraged touching the face, so the virus could pass into the mouth or nose more easily. The Covid symptoms I listed for the viewers were: cough, high temperature, shortness of breath; anything else, like a blocked nose, indicated an upper respiratory infection – nothing to worry our increasingly stretched healthcare services with. I felt reassured. Derek had none of the symptoms we were being warned about.

Yet when I came home from work that day and rushed upstairs to check on him, something about the look in his eye – fear, I think – hit me in the pit of my stomach. It was as though a full-scale battle was going on inside him. And it was clear he was losing the fight, even though he tried to hide how sick he was, so as not to worry me.

I couldn't get through to 111, so I rang Dr Hilary, who did a few short breathing tests on the phone with Derek and then told him to pass the receiver to me. 'Call an ambulance – do it now – and pack a bag for him. You know, just in case they need to admit him,' he said, trying to sound casual and reassuring.

There then followed a whirlwind, with me trying to 'keep things normal', like a cheerful actor in a sped-up 'Keep Calm and Carry On' public information film that I'm sure fooled nobody. I chattered away, trying to hide my fear and reassure Derek; I ran around, trying to tidy up and make the place look 'sorted', clearing a path for the paramedics, without knowing what kind of access they might need. I was trying to control a situation that was uncontrollable. Trying to think what to pack – Derek had only been to hospital once before, and never overnight. He was trying to reassure me, in turn; he was worried about the kids and telling me to keep them downstairs.

The ambulance seemed to take forever, but actually arrived in well under an hour. Earlier that day, on *GMB*, I had been reading out warnings that ambulances and hospital wards everywhere were in danger of being overwhelmed; we were being discouraged from calling for anything other than an extreme emergency. I worried that we might be taking an ambulance away from someone who needed it more. And with every minute that passed, I clung to the thought that if someone else needed it more, he couldn't be as ill as I feared.

The ambulance arrived and the paramedics came in, wearing plastic bibs and masks, and immediately put a mask on Derek. They pricked his finger to test his blood oxygen levels, which they said were dangerously low. They immediately swapped the PPE mask for an oxygen mask and mini oxygen tank. He said he was breathing fine and didn't have a cough. 'Well,' they said, 'the oxygen in your blood is low and you need to get to hospital urgently.'

This was before instant Covid tests were available, so

there was no way they could know for sure. But it was clear they thought he had it and feared he had it badly.

The two female paramedics were small, and Derek said he could walk unaided down the stairs to the hall. But then he stumbled, so they used a contraption to help him down, half-sliding him, half-pulling him downstairs. It was ungainly and comical, and at any other time he and I would have been in fits of laughter.

The kids heard the kerfuffle and came into the hall, despite my attempts to keep them away. As soon as he saw them, Derek pivoted away from his own distress and pain and leapt into reassurance mode. Being a dad and comforting the kids took priority over everything for him.

'Hi you two, I'm still not feeling that good, so these nice paramedics are taking me to hospital to make me better. Mum is going to stay here to look after you ...' They rushed forward to give him a hug. 'Better not,' he said, trying to sound as calm and jovial as he could. 'We don't want you catching this, do we?'

But nothing was going to stop them following him outside, eyes like saucers, solemn faced, as the paramedics hoisted him onto a stretcher and put an oxygen mask over his face. 'Look, it's like scuba diving,' he said to them, trying to make everything seem fun and fine. Then to me, more urgently, hissing, 'Take them inside!'

'Come on, let's go in. It's cold,' I said, ushering them back into the house.

I wanted so much to get into the ambulance with him, to hold his hand and reassure him. I knew he was terrified, fearing it might be the dreaded Covid, but also because he had never spent a night in hospital, never even been particularly sick with *anything*. He looked at me wild-eyed from under the oxygen mask, his face distorted beneath its elephantine plastic curves; then, as they shut the ambulance door, out of the kids' sight he pulled the mask off for a second, his eyes boring intensely into mine, heaving as much love and conviction my way as he could.

'This is not the last time you will see me, understand that, Kate ... I love you.'

The ambulance door was hurriedly shut and it sped away. He was gone. My loud, loving, rambunctious, utterly infuriating and utterly brilliant husband, leaving me standing on the pavement on a cloudy spring night, under a million invisible stars that I hoped would emerge to illuminate his journey to hospital and shine on him with all the magical healing power of the universe.

Gone forever. *That* Derek never came home.

And so began a 373-day fight for life that, in many ways, still goes on today. From the moment that door slammed, Derek's life hung in the balance – and with it my life and our kids' lives were held in suspended animation.

I felt as if I was holding my breath: I counted each second he stayed alive as a victory; telling myself if he could just get through this hour, this day, this week, there was a chance that he could come home. A chance for him to still be a dad, still be a husband; a chance for this whole nightmare to be something we could move on from; even a chance that one day in the future we could look back and see this as simply a terrible time we had all lived through. Something that might fade from our memories, that we could consign to history. I think the whole country was wishing the same – about Covid.

It didn't seem real, did it? It's hard to remember now how shocking those early news reports seemed about an invisible, incurable disease that was forcing people in foreign lands to stay inside. Lockdown. That could never happen here, we said. No one would put up with it. But it was coming for us – an unstoppable force. Never mind what we believed or disbelieved. We thought we lived in a safe, controlled world, where even cynics might expect our leaders and experts to protect us from global chaos, but Covid ran roughshod over us all, unleashing fear on a scale that no one of my generation or younger had ever felt before.

For the first time, I wondered if this could have been a tiny flavour of what my great-grandfather must have felt as he froze in a wet trench in France in the First World War. Looking down the line at the other men – boys, really – all scared out of their wits, with no idea whether they would see another day.

I thought about my grandmother, isolated in England,

where she had come to train as a teacher when the Second World War broke out. Her whole family were back home in Guernsey, under Nazi occupation, and she was unable to contact them to find out whether they were alive or dead. She would run to the stationery cupboard in her classroom to hide her fear from her pupils, her body shaking uncontrollably whenever bombers flew overhead. After a particularly bad phone call from the hospital, as I closed and bolted the door of my bathroom to hide my tears and fear from my children, I tried to channel her strength, and think about what had kept her going when she had no power to keep her loved ones safe or find a way to be with them.

Was this how my father felt during the Second World War, aged eight, as his mum and dad cuddled him, trying to distract him while they took shelter under the stairs? They lived close to London and they worried that Nazi bombers flying overhead, back to Germany, would drop their unused bombs, obliterating whatever lay beneath. I wondered if my children felt the same as my dad had done, comforted by his mother's hugs, but still seeing the fear in her face and sensing this was something she couldn't wish away with her usual, 'It's all fine, duckie.' I wondered whether my attempts at covering my fear might be as unconvincing, as unsettling, for my own kids.

The Blitz spirit was often mentioned during the early days of the pandemic. People from that generation remembered their parents taking in whole families whose houses had been bombed, neighbours sharing tiny slivers of butter (which was worth its weight in gold), and blackout parties with mass singalongs while V2s dropped overhead. People were terrified, but they put on a brave face and came together. In the pandemic, though, we were banned from contact outside our bubbles, could find no comfort in hugs, no reassuring grasp of a hand or light touch on an arm to say, 'I'm with you.' As people started to die in huge numbers, an elderly man who had lived through the Blitz in London as a child told me that the pandemic was almost worse, because the enemy was invisible, mysterious. 'At least we knew who we were fighting during the war,' he said.

The authorities clearly wanted to ignite that Blitz fighting spirit, which they hoped we all still had inside us, handed down from the war generation, a spirit that would help us come together and work through this. When you are following orders for the common good, you feel united against a common foe, and that engages a community spirit. 'Stay home – save lives – protect the NHS' even sounded like those wartime instructions: 'Loose talk costs lives'.

In 2020, our healthcare workers were our frontline troops, fighting a new foe that confounded all their medical experience, putting their own lives at risk, and often losing them. One of the worst errors of those early months was the decision to let untested patients be discharged from hospitals into care homes. This led to the generation who lived through the Second World War becoming some of the earliest casualties of mistakes made by the generation they had fought for.

I tried to think how the generations before us had coped with the uncertainty, the not knowing and the fear. My grandfather had told me they just had to follow instructions to the letter, and trust that the battle had some meaning and what they were doing was right. Despite the misery and the slaughter, they were readied to make the sacrifice because they had a purpose. It was hell, no doubt, and if they let their focus slip for a second, if for a moment they felt that the sacrifice wasn't for the greater good (a duty they'd been put on Earth to endure for a reason), the fear became too great. It froze them to the spot.

Each day, he would force himself to think of the war as just temporary, something to be endured; something that, if they all tried hard enough and followed instructions from 'above', they might just survive. 'Life became very bright,' my grandfather said, 'dazzling, almost, because we knew it could be taken away at any moment.' Then he looked me hard in the eye: 'Remember, Katy, where there is life there is hope.'

This simple thought, which encapsulated so much, struck home for me even as a child. I was reminded of it in those first weeks, after they had put Derek in an induced coma to keep him alive. It was comforting to think it might be my late grandfather talking to me, his presence still there in those lonely lockdowns when we were all stranded in our own homes. When for us, *our* home, the heart of comfort, felt so terrifying in Derek's absence, and was suffused by the fear that he might never come back.

I kept that vital thought with me when calls from the hospital came at random times, whenever the poor exhausted staff had a second to step away from saving lives to update terrified family members and let them know if their loved ones were winning or losing the battle. My first question, when they called, was always 'Is he still alive?'

I couldn't take in anything else until I'd heard them say 'Yes'. Because if the answer was no, in my head whatever information was coming next wouldn't matter. I was one of the lucky ones who got a yes; millions of others would be hearing a life-crushing no. And even with the yes, it took me a second to settle, to absorb it. Then I would say, 'Okay, go,' as new information was fired at me – vital details I needed to take on board so that I fully understood where Derek was in his battle to stay alive.

Even at other, quieter times, I'd repeat the phrase. It became my anchor. 'Where there is life, there is hope,' I would say to myself, over and over. Until it ran in my head like a song, a comforting lullaby – keeping me going, keeping a dream alive. I focused on it. I super-charged it in my mind so that it turned from a wish, or a dream, into a living hope: the light at the end of a very long tunnel.

'Manifesting', my friend Vickie calls it. 'Eyes on the horizon' is my mum's old-school equivalent. She would say this whenever a boyfriend had dumped me, or something hadn't gone my way, if a kid had been mean to me in the playground or, later, if I'd been passed over for a job at work. 'They will have their own reasons for why they are behaving like this,' she'd say. 'As long as you stay kind, positive and hardworking, you will win through.' I guess both are about positive thinking. Look forward, focus on the good, be grateful for what you have – don't give in to fear; push away negative thoughts, like fear, revenge and bitterness. And work like crazy on the things you can change.

Piers Morgan's version of this advice was to say to me, 'Garraway, treat this as the biggest story of your life. Your mission is to save Derek: research his state like you would a story, focus on it – push everything else to one side; think of it like you're on air and a big story is breaking.'

This advice helped, because it flipped me into professional mode. I could immediately harness skills that were familiar in a world where everything had become strange and nightmarish. And I knew that if I focused every brain cell on finding answers, there would be no space left to fret about the future. Diving deep into this story would stop my thoughts spiralling and hopefully ease the grip of fear.

So that's what I did. I started with Google and

followed research leads, drawing on years of experience and training to drill down and reach out for information. I made contact with doctors and anyone who looked as if they could help; I chased recommendations all over the world, trying to get my head round this thing called Covid.

Little was known when Derek went into hospital, other than that Covid could cause acute respiratory failure. It's hard to overstate what the medical profession was up against in the beginning. During Derek's first few days in hospital, one doctor told me on the phone: 'He is hanging in there; he's struggling but we don't think he needs to go on a ventilator. Not yet, at least, which is good, because we only have a limited number of ventilators, and our need has gone through the roof. In fact, not only are we struggling to find ventilators, unbelievably, we are in danger of running out of oxygen to run through them. I have been up all night trying to get more supplies and I think we are there. But everyone is in the same boat.'

My brain whirred as he was speaking: 'Christ, Derek might need a ventilator? But he doesn't need one *yet*. But they're considering it. Oh God, what if he needs one and there isn't one available?'

The fear surged and the thoughts spiralled.

I took a deep breath. 'Okay, what to do? What to do? I *have* to do *something*.'

I called everyone I knew, until a friend put me onto

another friend, who passed me to another friend, who had a friend who was a nurse in Kent. She got onto the NHS network and found out that the closest ventilator not in use in London was in Bromley.

Looking back, it seems mad – and arrogant. Did I really think I would be any better at finding ventilators than the authorities?! But I just couldn't bear to do nothing. When the doctors rang later that day to update me, I almost didn't say it. I was worried they might think I was interfering, or doing something unethical, trying to pull a fast one. But at the end of our conversation, I said, 'Look, just in case you are still struggling to find ventilators, there are some on the system in Bromley; there is less pressure on Kent right now.'

To my surprise they were delighted. 'Thank you *so* much,' they said. 'We'll pass it to logistics.'

I have no idea whether they used the information or if it benefited Derek. In the end, he wasn't put on a ventilator at that point, but I like to think it might have helped someone in need. And the mere fact that they were appreciative, and didn't laugh me out of court, showed me just how desperate they were. Any help was welcome. Without realising it at the time, this message lodged in my head: do what you can do to help, anything practical that takes you away from the torment and worry in your mind. Knowing all the while, of course, that it was the medics who offered the only real hope of saving Derek.

Then I started searching for medication, looking up the latest ideas on the internet. This was before vaccines or any treatment, before the vaccine trials had even started or President Trump had suggested drinking bleach. My research helped me to gain knowledge and feel like I was getting a little bit ahead of the game.

As time went on and lessons were learned, the goals changed. At first, the doctors said that survival was all about the lungs, because respiratory failure was causing the majority of deaths. Even though Derek's kidneys had failed and he was on dialysis, even though his liver was malfunctioning and his heart was in trouble, the doctors said the priority was getting his lungs working because if they couldn't get enough oxygen into his body it would be 'all over'. He was losing the battle against Covid so they decide to put him in an induced coma and onto the ventilator.

With Covid pneumonia, the lungs stiffen with infection and inflammation, so you literally can't breathe in or out. One doctor said Derek's lungs were 'locked solid' with Covid and it was 'a blessing' that he was in a coma; otherwise, he would have felt as if he was drowning, as if every breath was ripping his lungs apart. Covid restrictions prevented me from witnessing the horror. I couldn't see the wrenching, tortuous, barely-there movement of his lungs in and out but I could imagine it. Until that conversation, every time the nurse held the phone up to his ear, I had prayed he could hear me and feel the love I was sending him. But now, with the doctor's words in my mind, I desperately hoped in one way he felt nothing. I shuddered, too, thinking of what Covid was doing to his lungs, and what would be left of them afterwards.

Over the next few days, though, the doctors felt they were losing the battle. Even in the coma and on the ventilator, his oxygen levels were dangerously low. In my research I discovered they were using a piece of kit called ECMO that had previously mainly been used to support transplants and an Australian doctor contacted me to say they had found some success with this for Covid patients. The machine works by drawing blood out of one leg, oxygenating it and then putting it back into the other leg. This would take Derek's blocked-up lungs completely out of the loop and maintain oxygen flow around his body to keep his organs alive.

I spoke about this with the head of the unit and he said they had started trialling this technique with some patients here in the UK. It was high risk, though, because being on the machine traumatises the body and blood vessels, and doctors had found that patients could generally only cope with being on it for 21 days, at most. So we were praying for his lungs to recover in that time; otherwise there would be little hope. As each day passed, we had a terrible countdown, praying for signs of the infection retreating and the lungs starting to work. T minus 21, 20 … 10, 9 … but what would happen at T?

On day 21, with still no change, I begged the doctor on the phone, 'Please don't take him off the machine.'

'You are clear about that, are you?' he asked.

'Yes,' I said. 'Please, he is fighting, I know he is.' Then, quickly, 'It won't do him any harm, will it? I mean, no more harm than has already been done.'

'Hard to say really,' the doctor replied. 'But one thing is for sure: if you turn it off then he will die, because it's the only thing keeping him alive.'

Then why would we even consider switching it off? I felt a wave of panic. 'Is he trying to say there's no hope – is it *that* conversation?'

I tried to divine what his words really meant, to read beyond his measured, calm tone.

Then guilt kicked in. 'Are they trying to free up the machine for someone they think they have more hope of saving?' I asked myself.

I waited – was that a sigh?

'If you genuinely want that, then we will put it on his notes and keep going,' he said. 'But, you know …' There was another pause. 'There does sometimes come a point when you have to accept, Mrs Draper, that there is nothing to be done.'

It was the first time that word 'accept' had cropped up and my adrenaline was pumping so fast that it barely registered. Accept? Accept what – giving up, while there is still life? Accept letting go, when he is still breathing, fighting, struggling to come back to us?

The word scorched into my head and out the other side like a bullet. And the guilt and confusion it caused each time it slammed through me became harder to resist.

Later in the pandemic, I found out that people were staying on ECMO machines for weeks and months longer than doctors realised was possible in its previous use. Suddenly, miraculously, their lungs, like Derek's, began to work. Even destructive, knowledge-defying Covid could throw up a medical positive sometimes, when doctors, experimenting in dire circumstances – because why not, if it might save a life that would otherwise be lost? – discovered something new, even groundbreaking, through treating early Covid patients like Derek.

King Charles (at that time still Prince Charles) wrote me a sweet letter saying that if I ever needed a second opinion, he would be very happy for me to speak to his personal physician. It was much later, but I did it anyway, and the physician said they had since learned that I'd done the right thing by keeping Derek on ECMO, which was very reassuring.

Then one wonderful day, weeks after they feared it would never happen, Derek's lungs seemed to respond. It was time to wake him up out of his coma. I was dizzy with the possibility that everything might just be okay. Only … he couldn't wake up. What fresh battle was this? Was he going to be trapped forever in a comatose state? I thought the fight was about living or dying, but now there was a dreadful third option – being trapped forever. How could we fight this? How could we rescue him? I felt like the prince, hacking his way through the brambles, trying to reach Sleeping Beauty, when she and all the servants in the castle had been bewitched.

Love somehow found a way into the castle: the kids and I talked to him on FaceTime. We recorded messages from his friends and played them down the phone; our voices seeped through cracks in the stonework, breathing warmth into silent, icy halls; trying to bring him back to life and the world.

Where there is life, there is hope, and slowly Derek began to emerge from his long sleep. We were warned it wasn't possible to tell if he would even know us, but it was a start. Not yet time to open the champagne, but maybe we could put it in the fridge.

It was around this time that the news seemed to be full of stories about people coming out of hospital – patients who had been written off but who had got better and were being clapped by smiling NHS staff as they left. There were reports of miracles, too: the 93-year-old woman who had survived when Covid had ripped through her care home; the GP who said her final goodbyes to her husband and daughter and then recovered.

I longed for a miracle. I prayed that one day it would be Derek being clapped out of hospital. Every step of the way, we wanted him home. It was what we constantly longed for – our brains were trained on it. I'd had dreams of him standing and walking, being helped along – with the children by his side – still weak but absolutely himself: thanking the doctors, weeping with emotion, breathless but brilliant and finding just the right words to sum up the moment, just as he always used to. Like the final scene in a TV movie, he would stand on the doorstep of our house, hugging the three of us as the title credits rolled.

But I knew this outcome was still out of Derek's reach. He couldn't stand or hug us, even if he knew who we were. He couldn't really move at all; and when he did, he grimaced in pain. He only spoke a few words: a whispered 'yes' or 'no' and often 'I don't know.' Or just a blank stare.

Coming home seemed impossible, he was just too sick and frail, but I still believed we had to try. If we could only get him home, we could shower him with love, and maybe that would help us pull him out of his prison.

I knew I couldn't mend his body – the brilliant medics were working on that – so my next step would be to find a way of making our home suitable for him. We had to believe that Derek lying there blankly, paralysed, wasn't 'the end of the movie' – that it was just a cliffhanger in a long film. Feeling there was even the slimmest chance spurred me on, and spurred me on with renewed purpose. So I now had to think about the practicalities of him coming home. I just followed the principle from the movie *Field of Dreams*: 'If you build it, they will come.'

'I have to will this into existence,' I thought, even

though it seemed so unlikely. 'Prepare the way, put in the effort and believe; then it will happen.'

The changes to the house would be hugely expensive but it felt as though it was worth spending any money we'd saved and even going into debt because this was our family's greatest immediate need. What was the point of having money for a rainy day when you were caught in the middle of a storm? I guess now it might seem irresponsible but I had to believe that Derek would come through this, that he and I would get back to work and we could recover – we just had to get through this crisis.

Whatever the future held, I accepted that Derek wouldn't be walking when he came home. In fact he might still not even be able to sit up so we had to reconfigure the downstairs of our house to accommodate the width of a wheelchair, a stretcher, a hospital bed plus large pieces of kit like a hoist. Our doorways were clearly too narrow and needed to be widened; we needed a place to wash him downstairs, a wet room; and our sitting room would have to become his bedroom; so we would have to turn the kitchen into somewhere much more than just a place to cook.

People ask me how we coped during those days of not knowing Derek's fate from one hour to the next, when my head was full of questions: Will he live? Will he die? Please, God, no. What can I do about it? On one occasion I was actually told that he was dead, before finding out later that they'd got the wrong name and he was still alive.

Well, love got me through – the love I was sending Derek every second of every minute, and the love and support that was coming my way from friends, family and caring viewers. Sometimes this was a simple text with a love heart when I needed it most, other times it was practical. My friend Tonia Buxton, who is the face of the Real Greek Company, left plated-up dinners for me and the kids on the doorstep and texted us to let us know they were there. Rob Rinder would text me every morning to ask what we needed and my responses would range from Granny Smith apples (Bill's favourite) to Blu Tack, which definitely confused him! He texted back to say he hoped the Blu Tack wasn't some Trump-like cure for Derek we were experimenting with – it was in fact just to put some pictures up! Distraction for the children was vital and Laura Tobin focused on the morale of the kids, sending us things like doughnut-making kits – the arrival of her parcels always prompted squeals of delight.

Neil Thompson, my editor, happened to ring just an hour after Derek went off in the ambulance, with some very wise words. 'Don't focus on yourself or even on Derek,' he said. 'You can't do anything to make yourself feel better – you can't even help Derek right now – but you *can* help the kids. You are the one person who can make them feel stable, so let that be your focus.'

I did everything I could to help Bill and Darcey through

the trauma of their dad being so poorly. It was intense for them – for all of us – because he had the disease we were all shielding from in our homes, so the fear was everywhere. In the same way that working like crazy to help Derek pushed aside my ever-mutating worries, focusing on the children took me away from myself and my thoughts about what would happen to me.

But dividing my time between frantic research and looking after the children meant roping in the help of another friend – adrenaline. If you've ever spent a prolonged period of time under great stress, you'll know adrenaline is a faithful companion that keeps you in a constant state of 'fight or flight'.

Adrenaline is actually a wonder drug, so it's easy to understand why people become addicted to it. Also known as epinephrine (so good they named it twice), it's a hormone that regulates different bodily functions and is secreted by the adrenal glands to make everything in your body go faster, from circulation and breathing to metabolism.

Adrenaline increases blood flow to your muscles and your brain, which – along with a rise in blood sugar levels – gives you a surge of energy; it widens your pupils to let in more light; it relaxes the airways and gets you shallow breathing to allow more energy into your body. It's effective in so many ways. Your body is on high alert and you can stay awake, feel no pain and be quick-witted and responsive. Basically, it turns you into the Hulk –

without the anger issues. People surging with adrenaline have been witnessed performing extraordinary feats, such as single-handedly lifting a car to release a child trapped beneath it.

Yes, adrenaline has magical powers. Adrenaline is what kept the NHS workers functioning, with masks embedded in their faces as they worked 12- and 18-hour shifts and way, way beyond. It allows you to make fast decisions without thinking about long-term consequences. Those decisions are usually about weighing up odds and balancing risk in the long and short term; but when adrenaline is flowing, the issues are clear-cut. It's all about the present moment, life or death; there's no room for grey, no room for next year or even the next day. It's simply about survival, right now. Derek needs wider doors – pay for it. Never mind what that money was actually saved for, or what the consequences might be. The kids need time just to be cuddled to soothe their fears. Fine – schoolwork can wait. This was about surviving now, in the moment, because we genuinely feared we might not get another chance.

It felt at the time as though the government was also in an adrenaline-fuelled state, and making similar rapid, clear-cut decisions, for better or worse. They threw money at PPE and vaccines (successfully with the latter); and they provided lockdown furloughs that would keep people alive and afloat but have dire long-term economic consequences – and yet the furlough scheme seemed a better option than people breaking lockdown and risking everyone's safety by going out to earn money to feed their families.

And the cost of making decisions in this short-term, adrenaline-fuelled way? Well, I think we can see it all around us, can't we? Millions suffering from mental burnout, including children who lost out on schooling and a sense of self, and older people who were tipped into dementia by the isolation. Of course, those decisions were made to meet the short-term emergency but they have consequences. The list seems endless: the mental health epidemic unfolding among all ages; lower levels of trust in governance than before; the economic devastation impacting everybody's lives for the worse. Whatever mistakes we think the government may have made, on a human, individual level it may explain why they were in the state of mind to take risks.

While your adrenaline is pumping, you can only focus on the present. If you're bleeding out with a puncture wound, you can't worry about how deep and ugly the scar will be – you've got to heal the wound now and worry about the rest later. And that's how many of us were living during the pandemic. Maybe there was no other choice. It certainly felt as if there was only one option for our family. Survive.

But what about the long-term physical effects of living on adrenaline? I'd made good use of it while focusing on Derek's health, looking after the kids and going back to work – and, even though I didn't know it then, I was going to rely on it for a good while longer. However, like every other performance-enhancer, adrenaline has a negative impact on your body in the long term. It can lead to problems with metabolism, the heart, blood pressure, digestion, hormone balance, sleep, memory and concentration, headaches, anxiety and depression.

It can also tire out the glands that produce it – the adrenal glands that also release cortisol to help keep you going if you're in fight-or-flight mode for more than a short time. Cortisol is a natural steroid, and steroids are incredible. Ask any bodybuilder or someone who has asthma or arthritis and may actually need to take them from time to time. Yet you can't stay on steroids for too long – your skin gets thinner, your bones weaker, your blood pressure higher and you're at greater risk of infection and mood swings. Nor can your body keep pumping out adrenaline and cortisol forever without cost. It's like blood: if you give a pint of blood, your body will have replenished it within 24 hours (miracle!). But if a puncture wound isn't staunched, you will bleed to death.

I knew I needed to come off adrenaline at some point, even though it was what was then keeping me going: working day and night, living on my wits and loving Derek and the kids as hard as I could, longing for the moment Derek could come home.

Chapter 3

Poised

The longing went on and on. Every bit of the house felt as if it was bristling with expectation. We were as ready as we could possibly be – and now just waiting for the word from the hospital. But it was complicated.

There were big decisions to be made. The specialists obviously knew that Derek was nowhere near able to look after himself or be looked after just by me. He still needed intensive 24-hour care and couldn't do anything for himself, or even reliably communicate his basic needs. But they were also concerned that spending over a year in hospital – being cared for by strangers in full PPE – wasn't helping either. The neuropsychologist said he seemed to be regressing, retreating inside himself, struggling more and more, even though there were no further infections at this stage. They noticed he only really seemed to respond when the kids or I were on FaceTime, or when one of them tried to talk to him.

On top of the physical damage, it was also known that Covid had an emotional impact. Doctors in Italy were reporting that many of their hospitalised, surviving, severe Covid patients were displaying symptoms of post-traumatic stress disorder. They were recording severe depression too and, of course, emotions like survivor's guilt and shock. The neuropsychologist in charge of Derek said he was likely to be suffering all of these, on top of any neurological damage, and that keeping him in the alien, isolated world of a hospital ward wasn't helping his disengagement. So, a balance had to be struck between his emotional welfare and keeping him safe, and making sure he had daily access to the physio and occupational therapy that he needed to increase his strength and help him progress.

The debate raged between the specialists for weeks, and then we were told that Derek had run out of his NHS time allocation for recovery and there was a limit to funding further rehab or treatment. This really frustrated the medical team, as they said the whole point of our health service was to give care for as long as it's needed. They were exasperated by pressure on healthcare management to impose restrictions when it came to a disease as new as Covid, because they simply had no way of classifying Derek's situation or how long he needed. It's much easier to budget for conditions like stroke and cancer, I was told, with a recognised treatment pathway and a trajectory of expected recovery. I could understand that, but it was tragic for Derek, as he was already at the wrong end of an unknown disease with an impossible diagnosis, and I feared for the consequences of not extending his inpatient recovery.

We faced similar challenges when we were trying to convey what Derek would need in terms of nursing support and medical help if he came home. There was meeting after meeting online, as Covid rules meant we still couldn't meet in person, and we kept trying to explain to social care administrators just how Covid had affected Derek. The specialists were amazing and showed immense patience, but I remember when one *very* senior doctor, who never usually raised his voice, finally cracked.

The administrator had kept on insisting: 'We have a lot of experience with long Covid and we find that when patients get home, they feel much better. I bet you'll find that he suddenly gets up and walks and is back to his old self in no time. He might just be being a bit lazy – people do get like that, you know, when they have been in hospital for a long time.'

She said this last bit with what I assume was supposed to be a comforting wink.

'If only that could be true,' I thought.

But before I could savour even the fairytale possibility of it, the poor senior doctor finally lost it.

'Look, you can't possibly have *a lot* of experience with long Covid because we barely understand what this disease does at its height, let alone the after-effects, as it's only months old. And second, by the way, Derek's case is *not* long Covid as you think of it; it's a total medical catastrophe – on a scale my colleagues and I in the European forums have not seen. So, *no*, someone popping in a couple of times a day will *not* be enough and, *yes*, 24-hour care *is* needed.'

'God bless him,' I thought, little knowing that, once home, these frustrating conversations would become my daily life. Not that I blamed the administrator – she had no idea. It was all so new, and every element of the social and healthcare service was scrambling to cope, and still is, I fear.

In the end it was Covid itself that stepped in and made the decision, convincing the experts that home would indeed be best. The hospital had a Covid outbreak on Derek's ward and, because Derek was so vulnerable, they needed to move him but couldn't transfer him to another ward because of the risk of spreading infection. They also had to stop therapists coming onto the ward – it was effectively locked down – so he was just left lying in bed with two nurses keeping him safe. This was the moment to take the leap. I got a phone call to say 'We're on', and suddenly it was happening – after weeks and months of waiting and hoping and praying.

So much needed to be arranged just for the actual journey home. An ambulance wasn't available and, as this wasn't an emergency, not really justifiable, so I researched with the occupational therapist (OT) the best kind of private mobility vehicle. They didn't have one available at short notice that could take a stretcher, so we opted for one where he could sit up in an ultra-supportive wheelchair. When he had first arrived at that hospital, he had been in a full coma; and even though he was doing much better on the ward at supporting his own head with his neck muscles, no one wanted to take any chances with his first journey.

We then had a week, which felt like being in a First World War trench, waiting for the call to go over the top. Was it on, this morning? No, it had to be put back until they got approval after visiting the house to inspect the changes we'd made – on, off, on, off …

At home, we were scrubbing and disinfecting every-thing in sight.

We still had Covid restrictions at this point and the virus remained rife, so Derek's parents didn't feel it was safe to travel down to be there when he arrived. But I wanted Derek to have someone to greet him, not just me, and to support the children while I went to the hospital, letting me focus on Derek. So my parents arrived and began putting up 'welcome home' banners, which they made with the children, even though it almost felt like tempting fate after waiting this long. We still had the one that the kids had made in spring 2020 – now very faded – but I said, 'Put it up. This is our moment, whatever the future holds.'

Day after day, I went to the hospital, only to be told, 'It can't happen today', and then I'd ring the kids and say, 'Not today.'

So by the time I went in on Wednesday, 7th April, I had managed my expectations to the point that as I sat in reception, filling in forms and waiting for the nurses and the hospital administrators to say it couldn't happen, it was almost a shock when eventually a supervisor appeared and said, 'Yes, it's on!'

I felt my heart race – this was it!

She led me into a back room for the obligatory Covid test, then I was dressed in full PPE to go to the ward. She took me up in a small staff lift. That way, she said, we wouldn't come into contact with anyone else, and we could minimise the chance of infection.

The lift felt frustratingly cranky and slow, or maybe it was just that my heart and head were racing so fast. Then suddenly the lift doors opened and, unbelievably, Derek was there, in front of me. It was such a shock to see him in his own clothes after more than a year of hospital gowns that for a second I couldn't take it in. He looked, well, he looked like Derek, the old Derek, albeit frail and pale and slumped awkwardly in the specialised wheelchair. I looked at him for a split second that seemed like hours, trying to take in what I was looking at, and then simultaneously we both burst into tears!

I knelt down in front of him so that we were at eye level and gently clasped both of his hands.

'This is *it* – you are coming *home*,' I said, looking him hard in the eyes.

He stared intently back, then through tears mouthed, 'Love you.'

Suddenly I was aware of the nurses and staff around him, who were all crying too, all talking at once, in sentences that floated over me. 'He didn't want to wait in bed', 'too anxious and excited', 'wanted to be ready to go', and 'knew he was coming home'.

I gathered myself and took in how wonderful the moment was.

Then I had to get back to the practical stuff. 'Are the physio and occupational therapist here? Does anyone know if the transport is ready?'

No, not yet – and of course there needed to be a handover.

Derek was breathing very hard and going pale and clammy. 'Right,' I said, 'I don't want to be a killjoy but I think we need to get you lying flat so you can rest while I go through the handover and then you'll be rested enough for us to take you home. We'll get you back up when the transport is here.'

He squeezed my hand hard and looked terrified.

'Don't worry, I am not going to leave you,' I said

firmly, returning his squeeze. 'This *is* happening. We are going home. Let's just get everything in order while you rest so that you have strength for the journey.'

A couple of hours later we were ready to go. We had bags of stuff that Derek had accumulated over the year he'd spent in various hospitals. There were Lego bits the kids had made, heartbreakingly sweet little tableaux of figures made to look like me, the grandparents, Darcey and Bill and, of course, in the centre their dad – at his desk, working away and smiling. They had even chosen his company's colours and put a psychotherapist's couch in the corner.

The nurses carefully wrapped them in tissue.

There were paintings and pictures, so he'd had something to look at on the bare walls; messages and photos from anyone we thought might get a reaction; an array of objects to trigger memories, including beach pebbles and crystals from his office desk that he could hold in his hand; large, brightly coloured banners from his office at home; the books he'd written; favourite soft toys from his childhood; photographs from family holidays; and pictures of friends from all the vivid chapters and stages of his life. As we placed them all in large suitcases, it felt as if we were packing a white elephant stall of his life and the love we all felt for him. It felt tragic but wonderful that he no longer needed them to inspire him in hospital, because he was coming home with the hope of *living* his life, rather than just looking at it, frozen memories dangling above his head.

There were so many large medical contraptions that we needed to transport (on top of all his bits and pieces) that I had to book a second cab, as we couldn't even begin to get them all in the mobility ambulance.

Then we got the green light! The transport was here.

Two physios helped us carefully move Derek back into the specialised wheelchair. The chair had a bar support going up the back of his spine and around his neck to support his head. He had started to do much better at holding his head up on the ward, but no one wanted to take any chances on London's bumpy roads.

Outside we hit a surprising obstacle: no one had realised just how tall Derek is, from his waist to the top of head. For his height – six foot two – he has surprisingly short legs! The length is all in the waist-to-head bit. This was something I used to tease him about all the time, saying he had the inside leg of a meerkat and the upper body of a giraffe.

'I come from a long line of pit ponies,' he'd retort. 'My legs may be stumpy but they'll never let you down.' Oh the irony, looking at their frailty now, thin enough to snap in the wind.

But even in his shrivelled state, when sitting propped upright, his upper body was so tall that they couldn't get him into the mobility vehicle without bending his head, which he couldn't safely do. And the physios were still worried about him bashing his head on the roof, should we hit a bump. The staff realised they had never seen him upright or attempted to move him, other than on a stretcher. We went back inside while they lowered the supports in the vehicle. I squeezed his hand. 'Not long now … they have forgotten you are the "big man".' He smiled weakly.

And we were off. With our slow-moving vehicle and the six-seater taxi behind, crammed with his stuff and all the kit and equipment he needed for the future, we looked like a mini-presidential convoy. Inside our 'limo' were the driver, an OT to oversee Derek, and me. Derek was at the back, the wheelchair secured with specialist locks and pulleys to minimise any shaking. I had a sliver of a seat to the side and slightly in front so that I could be near him. It was wonderful, as I was close enough to reach back and hold his hand.

As we pulled away, his eyes were wide and he was rigid. 'Is he ill?' I thought. 'Oh no, is he going to have a seizure?'

'Was he terrified?' No, it wasn't fear, it was something else.

'Are you okay?' I asked him.

He nodded. It was a tiny gesture, the merest of movements, but I caught it. It was like a satellite docking on a space station – I had come into his orbit.

Of course, how could I have been so stupid? I had been so focused on the practical aspects, going through all the processes to get him home – making our house safe for him, getting everything he needed at the hospital ready, going through all his medication, making sure he was physically safe and rested enough; like a horse with blinkers concentrating only on the road ahead, I hadn't allowed myself a second to think how he would *feel*. I knew he wanted to come home but hadn't considered the actual reality of the moment, how leaving the alien but protected world of the hospital would affect him. What would this massive change be doing to him mentally and emotionally?

His eyes stretched even wider, as if he was trying to take it all in, filter it and process it. Was he remembering? Was he terrified? Did he even understand what was happening? Was this an awakening, a new beginning, the light of the world shining brightly outside the entrance of solitary confinement? Or was it like opening the door midway through processing a film, bleaching out the image?

I waited. Was he going to close his eyes, or faint? Would he try to shut it out, or shut down? No, he kept his eyes open and they grew wider and wider, sucking in the sights until he looked as if he would burst. Now I was getting scared.

'Are you okay?' I asked again, craning my neck round to try to make eye contact, feeling helpless. He moved his head; it wasn't so much a turn as a sort of winding a ratchet – barely a few degrees, but a definite, conscious movement.

'Is it just that it's very overwhelming?' I asked, stating the flipping obvious.

Derek blinked slowly like a cat, then started moving his mouth as if he was half-chewing, half-swallowing. It looked weird to me then because I hadn't seen it before – hadn't picked it up on Facetime – but I came to know that this was him gathering himself, trying to connect mouth to brain, connecting reality to the locked-in world he had been in. It seemed to be the most almighty effort. Then he stopped.

Had the battle inside him been lost? Or was I just imagining that he was trying to 'come out' at all? He grew glassy-eyed and very still.

'Is it very overwhelming?' I asked again.

'Of course.' Barely a whisper.

Now I was the wide-eyed one. Not just because it was more than a nod, or a yes/no accompanied by a blank stare that we'd had previously when trying to communicate, but because of the *tone* of voice. It was his 'old' tone. A connection, a 'normal' connection, like I was the buffoon to think otherwise, like he was surprised I was even asking. Maybe my sense that he understood more than he could express *was* right after all.

It was a flash of the old Derek, an echo that stirred so much hope.

'Yeah, of course it is,' I said. And gave his hand another squeeze.

As we moved through the streets, silence swept over

us – a thick, overwhelming silence that developed its own presence, a shadow self that was travelling with us – separating us and connecting us at the same time.

We were travelling very slowly, because we didn't know what Derek could tolerate in terms of movement, and I think the lovely OT felt a little bit awkward in the silence. She started making small talk, being nice, trying to be helpful.

I turned around to Derek and he was looking really, really stressed. 'Is this too much for you?' I asked.

And he said, 'Yes.'

I turned back to the OT. 'I'm really sorry. I think this is quite a big moment for Derek and maybe our chatter is too much.'

Derek squeezed my hand and mouthed 'Thank you.' I felt connected to him – I still knew what he needed. A rush of love – and relief – swept through me.

We carried on in silence; I couldn't take my eyes off him, watching his every flicker, searching for what any of it meant. Suddenly he looked at me, focusing hard, as if to say, 'Don't stare at me.'

'Is even me looking at you too much?' He nodded.

It was as if just being out in the world was intense enough and he couldn't take my gaze as well – he needed to absorb everything in his own way, at his own pace.

I turned to face forward and realised that I hadn't thought for a moment about our route or where we were. People were bustling around, shopping, laughing, chatting, grumbling, and everything seemed incongruously normal, while inside our vehicle everything was technicolour and life-changing. I wondered if it felt strange for Derek, too, that the world had been carrying on while he had been teetering on the edge of a cliff for so long. Had he even remembered that there *was* an outside world while he was locked in a sterile, white hospital ward, where nothing, neither his body, nor his mind, was normal?

Suddenly, as we started to climb a hill, I recognised where we were.

'Isn't the Tavistock along here?' I wondered out loud.

The Tavistock and Portman NHS Foundation Trust, a mental health centre based in north London, specialises in therapies for adults and children and has a long history as a centre for psychiatric research. Derek had a long-standing connection with the Tavistock and, before he got sick, had been elected as a governor there. It's an inconspicuous building (apart from the huge statue of Freud outside) and if you didn't know it was there you could easily walk past it without realising its importance. I was looking for the statue, forgetting that it had been covered up for cleaning and renovation, because I wanted to point it out to Derek, to help him get his bearings. But I suddenly realised I'd missed it and said, 'Oh, I think we've just gone past the Tavistock, haven't we?'

I turned to look at Derek. He was crying, actually sobbing. 'Did you spot it, did you see it?' I asked him and he nodded and mouthed 'Of course.' I couldn't believe it.

Obviously, it was very poignant because he was a world away from that person, the governor of the Tavistock and the mental health campaigner, but for me it was also a moment of massive elation. 'He has recognised the Tavistock!' I thought. 'That must mean he knows where he is. It means he remembers the Tavistock, what it means to him and his work there.'

It was just so huge, so enormous.

'Yes, of course you saw it,' I said, answering my own question. 'Did you see the statue?'

'No,' he said, 'it's covered up ... renovated.'

So he *had* actually spotted the building! It was just amazing because, until that moment, I wasn't sure he even remembered that he was a psychologist. Did he, like me, wonder whether he would be one again? That was too much. My mind was running away with me.

Back to focusing on the journey.

All the while, I had been keeping Bill and Darcey up to date. They were waiting at home with my mum and dad to greet Derek. Now I texted them to let them know we were on our way.

Looking up from my phone, I said, 'By the way, I'm not doing something random. I'm texting so that Darcey and Billy know where we are. As you can imagine, they are really excited to see you!'

He looked emotional. 'Good,' he mouthed.

We went through bits of London that were unfamiliar to me – to avoid as many speed bumps as possible,

I assumed. Then we were nearing our house. We live on a very, very long road, and we were approaching it from the far end.

As we got closer, I rang Darcey, but Bill grabbed the phone. 'Right, we're getting really close. Stand by and get yourself organised.'

Bill didn't even answer me; he just screamed, 'He's nearly here!' at the top of his voice, and I heard Darcey scream back.

'Are you okay?' I asked.

'Yes, Mum, of course. It's just like the best Christmas Eve ever. I'm so excited!'

I turned my focus back to Derek and gently said, 'I think we might be getting quite close now.'

He started crying and said, 'I know.'

'Are you upset because ...' I began, and before I could finish, he said, 'Thought never see again.'

'I know, I know.' The tears were welling up in my eyes now too.

It was just amazing – amazing that he could articulate it, both tragic and wonderful that he felt it.

We pulled up and, as always, there was no space for us to park very close to the house, but I could just see the kids looking out of the top window.

They immediately disappeared from view, running downstairs and out the front door.

It was taking quite a while to unstrap Derek and I kept on gesturing to the kids to stay back. I didn't want them to speak to him until he could see them, so that he could have that moment.

And then we were out and we turned him to face the children. Bill and Darcey jumped towards him and there was a massive hug and everyone was crying with joy. We came inside, where my mum and dad were crying too, but our tears were no surprise to any of us.

It was a strange moment as we came into the house. Everywhere you looked there was clear unmistakable evidence of how life had suddenly changed: the hospital bed, the mechanical hoist, widened doors, access ramps, the wet room replacing Derek's old familiar workshop. But so much that he was familiar with was still there. His Birkenstocks were by the front door where he had left them. His hat rack made out of the skull and antlers of a deer, adorned with his Panama hat and Darcey's riding hat – I'd objected to the rack, not liking the idea of a dead thing on the wall, but Derek had named it Siegfried and justified it by telling me that it was 'dead anyway', and that Winston Churchill had had one! So I gave in. And what was he seeing? The promise of family life again or the possibility that things might have irrevocably changed. I wondered what Derek was feeling.

Then the OT and the driver left. The door closed and it was just us. And all we could think of was the joy of him actually being there and I saw in his face that was what he was feeling too. It felt like this moment lasted hours, at least to Darcey and me, but actually it was just a few minutes. I realised I didn't quite know what to do next, so in a classically British way, I said,

'Would you like a cup of tea?'

He said, 'Okay.'

'One sugar, right?'

He nodded.

I made the tea but he didn't really drink it, because he couldn't hold the cup. It was just the ritual, a classic way of filling empty space. I held it up for him to sip. It was so overwhelming.

I then said, 'Have you noticed the changes? We've got really big doorways so that you can move around.'

'Yes,' he said. He was straining his head to try and look at something.

I just knew it was the fridge he wanted to see because it had been an ongoing source of light-hearted disagreement between us before he got sick. It had begun one morning when I was the first up and in a spring-cleaning mood. I must have been eager for the uncomplicated satisfaction that comes from creating shiny clean surfaces which, minutes before, were cluttered and chaotic – and the fridge door was an obvious target. Derek had long been in the habit of putting up photos and kids' drawings on the door and several years' worth of them were now patchworked across it, ink fading, edges curling. He was devastated when he came down to breakfast that day and found the door bare and gleaming, wiped down for the first time in years.

'That's my view every morning with my orange juice; my memories, my picture of our lives,' he said. He was so upset.

Chastened, I retrieved every tatty scrap of paper and under his instruction carefully put them back in the same place. After that, the fridge door gallery was sacrosanct, treasured. (And it's the last thing I'll ever mess with, given the scale of the other changes.)

'Don't worry, I haven't moved anything on the fridge door!' I said.

Was that a smile?

Then that was enough. I could see that he was flagging, pale and crumpled. This was the longest he had been upright in a sitting position since he'd got sick – and all the stimulation and emotion must have been exhausting for him.

'Do you need to lie flat?' I asked him.

A nod.

We got him into the newly kitted-out sitting room (now his bedroom) and used the mobile hoist to heave him onto the bed. Bill and Darcey were buzzing. 'Look, this is what we've made for you, Dad,' they said. 'You'll be comfy here until you are better.'

We sat watching him as he closed his eyes and disappeared into a deep, deep sleep. All these months of prayers and we were finally all home together! 'Oh God, he's here,' I kept thinking.

A tsunami of relief and gratitude washed over me.

This was what we had all prayed for, hoped for and tried to will into being. 'Everything has changed in the last hour and a half,' I thought, in amazement. '*Everything* has changed. He knows he's here. He knows Bill and Darcey, he knows me.'

So it felt wonderful. But I also realised that it was not the end.

I went into the kitchen and started laying the table for something to eat. 'Why aren't you laying four places, Mum?' Billy asked.

I had got so used to it just being three and, of course, I knew that Derek couldn't actually eat the meal with us, but somehow his question hit home. We were no longer three – we were four; we were back to the number of family members we were meant to be and we needed to start as we meant to go on. Whatever Derek's limitations, he was here, he was home, and we had to find ways of making that work.

So we did. I laid four places and we got him to the table, even though he needed to lie flat next to it, just propped up enough so that he could see us and be part of it; and then the kids and I sat down with him. I looked around this table that we had always eaten at, the kids' faces shining with delight that their dad was there, and Derek smiling back at us as best he could, beaming with joy and love as they talked to him. I realised that whatever changed, whatever the future held, we were together and we were a family again.

Chapter 4

Adapting

Derek was home, giving us a chance to restart and reshape our life together as a family. It was different, of course, because we were all scarred by what we had been through. Derek's damage was visible, and we all needed time to heal.

Having been given a chance that so many others had been denied, I felt determined to try to bring Derek back to us. We had to succeed, not only because we wanted it so desperately for *us*, but also out of a sense of duty to those who hadn't had the chance to even try. We had been told so many times it was a miracle he had survived at all and now we seemed to have a second miracle – he was *home* and we were euphoric with gratitude.

Together at last, as a family, we can do this, I resolved. There was a sense of optimism everywhere in the spring of 2021, wasn't there? The long, cold, dark winter without a Christmas, without families and friends to brighten it up, had passed. The agonising separations were over; the vaccine was available and seemed to be working; we were getting back out into the world that Covid had kept us all from, for so long. Life was moving again, after months and months on hold. People began returning to their places of work and seeing friends again – the novelty of that hadn't yet worn off. As for the realities of the economic crisis, the delays in NHS health treatments and the mental health cost, the full force of all that hadn't yet been felt.

'We might be battered and we might have changed dramatically,' was the feeling, 'but maybe we *can* get through this after all.'

The children were just so happy to have their dad home; it burst out of them and poured over him. He was here, he was real, not just a two-dimensional image on the iPad they'd had to use to talk to him in the hospital. When they were only able to connect with him on FaceTime there must have been times when he seemed like an illusion, or a hologram, never tangible enough for them to feel truly confident that he would be part of their lives again. Having him home solidified the hope of other things becoming real: of him getting stronger and better; and being their dad again in the way they wanted him to be.

The nervousness that had overcome them when they

first saw him and took in his emaciated frame – when they had stood back, scared he would break if they hugged him – had fallen away. Now when he held out an arm out to greet them, it was barely a movement, barely a gesture of his right hand, yet it was enough to unleash a tidal wave of love.

We couldn't say enough or do enough to express all the bottled-up emotions we had been holding back for more than a year – and neither could Derek. He cried and cried – happy tears – a mixture of relief and hope and, yes, pure love. He didn't want the children or me to leave him even for a moment. It was as if, when we weren't in his sight, he feared all this might just be a dream and he would wake up in the hospital again, surrounded by strangers in PPE.

He didn't have to worry; we didn't want to leave his side either. We didn't sleep a wink that first night, we hovered like new parents over their baby's crib, half-terrified half-ecstatic that something would go wrong – and consumed with an overwhelming sense of, now what?

I lay on the small sofa next to his 'hospital bed', listening to him breathe. With each breath I felt relief, and with the subsequent silence: panic! Sometimes I dozed off, then woke with a start, realising he had gone quiet; I'd spring up and lean over him, willing him to breathe in. And then he would, with a huge rasping gasp. Was this normal? Was this okay? Yes, he was breathing, but should he be stopping like that? As I took in the magnitude of the responsibility that caring for him at home was going to be, it dawned on me how much my role had changed from the moment he had been wheeled through our door.

Of course, I had felt a massive sense of responsibility for Derek from the second he was first whizzed away in the ambulance. And, just as I knew he would have done for me, I got stuck into finding out as much as I could about his condition and doing whatever I could to get help.

But this was different.

After more than a year at arm's length, mostly not being able to visit in person, it was magical to have him home ... but frightening too. Now all the extraordinary nursing and medical knowledge that I had marvelled at in the hospital, which had kept Derek alive, was no longer present. There would be no nurse popping in to take his blood pressure and check beeping monitors, no calm doctor at the end of a bleep, no scanners and tech at the ready to bring him back to life should his heart stop, and no on-site lab available day and night to test his blood, skin and urine for infection. I was the first line of defence against something going wrong – and there were countless things that could go wrong: from major organ malfunction to the ingress of a microscopic speck of bacteria, ten times smaller than a single cell. This last one, I knew, was a scary, stealthy enemy; Derek's double incontinence meant he was at high risk of skin and bladder infections, as well as chest infections that could spiral into a rapid decline in his overall health in a matter of hours. I had to be alive to every tiny change in Derek's state. It gave me a huge feeling of responsibility – and no little fear.

It was a massive step, from not being able to see him, from not even being able to speak to him on the phone initially; and also from the months when he was in a coma and we simply had to put our trust in the doctors who were looking after him. While he was in hospital, I'd been able to run around trying to get information and feed that information back to them. So I was still doing something. But this was different, now that *we* were doing the hands-on caring; still living from one minute to the next, trying to get our heads around how to keep him alive.

Of course, I'd been warned about the risks and responsibilities I would be taking on. When it was proposed that Derek should be released to be cared for at home, the doctors had sat me down to spell out what lay ahead. They made it very clear: Covid had ravaged him from the top of his head to the tips of his toes. Inflammation had rampaged through him, damaging his heart, his lungs, his liver and kidneys, his digestive system – every cell in his body, in fact. It had also spread throughout his brain and affected the nerve connections to all the muscles in his body.

Little was known about the effects of Covid on

anything but the lungs at this point, so the medics couldn't calculate how the damage might manifest in the long term. As the body is totally inter-connected, it wasn't really possible to work out what needed tackling first, nor even what the biggest threat was. When the Covid inflammation ran through Derek's brain, had that left damage that prevented him talking? Or was the difficulty in speaking a result of damage to the voice box itself, caused either by more Covid inflammation or by having a tracheotomy or tubes down his throat for months to breathe and feed?

Was he unable to communicate because of neurological damage, making the signals from his brain impossible for his body to react to? Or was he unable to move because his muscles had wasted away and his body was so weak? Or a combination of both? We weren't even sure he had fully emerged from the state of minimal consciousness that he'd spent weeks in after coming out of the coma.

Yes, he could react to noise and to us: he seemed reassured and delighted by us being there; and when he was startled by a noise our voices calmed him. Our love appeared to reassure him; but for us, used to the Derek we had known before, it was very hard to read how deep that went. He was extremely photosensitive. We had to keep the curtains closed; and if we turned the ceiling light on in his room to re-position him, he recoiled in horror, screwing his eyes up as if in pain. If more than one person spoke at a time or there were people shouting outside or if the TV volume was too high, he would grimace and we would have to turn everything off and let him 'power down', as I called it. Then, after a while, he seemed to gather himself, 're-boot', and be able to cope with moments, sometimes hours, of being more 'present', more aware. Was this state temporary or permanent? We just didn't know.

We were told there was a hole in his heart caused by Covid, but what effect was that having? His kidneys had failed and he had been on dialysis for a long time: they 'seemed' to be working now, but how well and for how long? And his liver had also been in distress. How long would that function? It wasn't possible yet to gauge how well each organ was working or how each individual organ's struggles were affecting the overall picture.

The only thing that would help us understand all this was time, I was told. And time – *with* him and *for* him – was something we had so desperately wanted, were so grateful to have and happy to give. But it was also overwhelming. I felt like a sentry in a constant state of high alert; guarding his life while the whirligig of assessment kept me in a state of permanent anxiety (adrenaline pumping), dominating my every waking minute and whispering worries in my ear while I tried to sleep.

We couldn't be confident that any part of his body was definitely working okay. As Covid is a relatively new disease, and scientists are still discovering its full effects, the doctors didn't know what the trajectory of recovery might be. This left us in a constant state of fear that, any minute, he might have to go back into hospital. At no point since he came home have we felt that he was now 'safe' and in recovery. And even the experts can't reassure us.

Even the simple act of breathing, the essence of life, felt precarious. He no longer needed the apparatus to breathe. He was off the ventilator. But clearly his lungs weren't functioning effectively. It looked so heavy and laboured as I watched him hauling oxygen in and out; it still does. It took the biggest effort and reminded me of an early combustion engine I saw powering up in a museum once as a kid, bellows and cogs slowing and juddering with every cycle, only just making it round to – exhale! – and repeat.

As I watched him, the doubts crept in. Had I finally gone completely mad? Had I placed us all in further jeopardy by taking on too much? Had I adapted the house to accommodate an insurmountable problem? Brought an unbearable pressure to bear on our family, on the kids, on me and yes, on Derek, too? The aim of bringing Derek home was to help him get stronger and bring him back to us, mentally and emotionally, as far as possible. But could I even keep Derek alive, let alone help him to thrive? Before we could even think about recovery, we had to succeed in simply keeping him safe.

'Oh my God,' I thought, in the still of the night. 'What on earth made me think I could do this?'

But then I thought about the hundreds of thousands – perhaps millions – of people all over the world doing exactly the same thing: caring for the ones they love, fearing for them, riding their fears and ploughing on. I imagined us linked by invisible bonds as we quietly enacted our tasks: the cleaning, wiping, dabbing, patting, washing, drying, fetching, carrying and changing; the speaking of words of tender reassurance. I felt our thoughts weaving themselves into a blanket of love, circling the world like a hug, easing the pain, offering comfort amid uncertainty and fear. And suddenly I felt less alone. Unlike Atlas, holding up the sky single-handedly for all eternity, there were many of us sharing this burden of care, each connected to the other by the thread of what truly makes us human – love.

I thought, too, of the millions of others who didn't have the chance to care for someone they loved – who would have envied me my fears, because they were facing a future *without* their loved ones.

'Okay,' I told myself, 'park your fears, focus on the love and the wonderfulness of him being home – let that drive you on.'

On the day Derek left hospital, I was handed a plastic bag containing his medication, box after box of it, dozens of blister packs, tubes and bottles.

'How do I know what medication to give him and when?' I asked. Being a desperate collector of facts (facts were always what I reached for to steady myself, the journalist in me probably), I had to ask what they were all actually for. 'Don't worry,' the discharge nurse said. 'You don't need to know what they are for; they're all prescribed by a doctor and there is a system for what to give and when. The hospital pharmacist will write to your GP, and they will issue instructions to Derek's carers.'

I didn't feel particularly reassured by this. It might have been instinct on my part or perhaps my lack of confidence was down to my experience of the past year, which had shown me that 'systems' don't always work as they should.

Then she added the ominous caveat, 'Or that is what is supposed to happen, anyway.'

Right, definitely not reassured – especially as I knew Covid had put an intolerable strain on an already overstretched system.

'Okay, we're going to have to go through this now, so at least I know what happens when. Because I have to be *you* now, don't I? It starts from today,' I said to the exhausted-looking nurse. 'You know, just in case,' I added, trying not to sound crushing.

It took two hours, largely because they had to check everything with the pharmacist, but thank goodness we did, because it took weeks for the official medication distribution kits – dosette boxes – to arrive.

Darcey found a clipboard among Derek's old work stuff, tied it to the bed and made daily charts with the timings for his medications so that we could tick off what we had given. It was a bit like playing nurse for her – obviously I had to supervise – but it gave her something practical to 'get involved with' and actually, as a system, it served us well.

I was still terrified of making a mistake, though, and I was constantly checking the correct dosage, popping tablets out of blister packs, and checking again.

Of course, as the days turned into weeks, people came in to support us. The carers arrived almost as soon as Derek got home. Every single carer was wonderful and their tenderness and devotion moved me so much that I'd frequently cry with gratitude when they arrived.

I didn't realise how little information carers are given before they arrive to look after someone until I experienced it. I really felt for them. In Derek's case it was understandable in a way, as he came out of hospital when Covid was still severely restricting who could be allowed in. Under normal circumstances, when the system is working as it should, the care manager comes in to be fully briefed and work alongside the hospital teams, so they can be trained in how to look after the individual patient. That is how it is supposed to happen, but the carers confided that it frequently – even usually – didn't. Usually I, too, would have been able to spend time at Derek's hospital bedside, learning how to care for him; but, due to a fresh outbreak of Covid on his ward, that didn't happen either. As it was, I'd only had a whistle-stop tour of the basics, and hoped the community nurses would be able to tell me more.

Now, when the carers arrived, they were given a half-page of notes beforehand, at best; and some arrived with no idea at all about Derek's condition or how to handle it. To be fair, Derek's case was so unusual that it was hard for anyone to truly brief them, but I quickly realised that in this new world of caring for him at home, I was suddenly the 'expert' because I was the only one who had been through Derek's Covid journey from the beginning.

As the first weeks stretched into months, there were often new carers for the day or night shifts, who needed to be fully briefed, which meant starting from the beginning every time. What if I missed something out – a crucial, lifesaving detail? It was terrifying. I realised that we needed some kind of continuity to keep him safe and begged to have regular carers, but it just wasn't possible for weeks, as they were so short-staffed. Derek's sudden discharge from hospital and the complications of his case made it even more challenging to find the right people to look after him.

Some carers arrived having only been told that he was suffering from the after-effects of Covid – 'long Covid', as it was beginning to be called – which back then people mostly saw as lung issues and breathing difficulties. Each was in a state of shock when they met Derek and saw him near-paralysed and unable to communicate, doubly incontinent too. Wide-eyed, they'd say, 'This can't be just Covid, surely? Was he paralysed before he got it?' It didn't seem possible to them that Covid alone had nearly wiped out a fit 50-year-old.

Even now, when we have a hospital visit, although we're often at the same hospital where he's been treated in the past, the departments are so specialised and segregated that they don't have his full information. For example, Neurology might have made a recommendation to the Autonomic Department to check out why his blood pressure might be so unstable and discover what else might be affecting his nervous system, but when you arrive to have the tests done, the full back history hasn't been passed over from one department to the other.

The staff, like the carers, disbelieve that the damage can only be caused by Covid, checking and rechecking their one page of notes and asking, 'But what else has done this, surely not just Covid?' Even when you go for an X-ray, again that's in the same hospital, even as part of the same visit, the radiographers are in disbelief, asking all the same questions. People are still not understanding, three years on, the devastation that Covid can cause generally, and the devastation to Derek in particular, and they always ask why he wasn't sent to them sooner, adding they could have helped more. I then have to explain that there was a delay in referrals and a breakdown in communication, and that it certainly wasn't from a lack of us pushing for it. They shake their heads and say, 'We're so sorry, it's a nightmare at the moment, we just can't do what we need to do.'

With even the most senior medical experts still trying to get their heads around it, it's not surprising that in those early weeks and months, when I'd helped with re-positioning Derek during the day, the carers would wake me up at night, to ask, 'Is this normal? Has he done it before? Can I just check what you do when he seems to be coughing to the point of choking?' And I was glad they did; I would much rather miss a bit more sleep than have guesswork lead to disaster.

As carers came and went, it was an adjustment getting used to having complete strangers in the house, especially for the children. When they were young, we'd never needed live-in nannies, even though I had left the house in the wee small hours for breakfast television all their lives. Derek was there for those shifts, getting them up and giving them breakfast; and when he worked late in the day, I would pick them up from school and do tea until he came home for bedtime stories and cuddles. The grandparents had always been around too, taking turns to come and stay with us in London and muck in, from when the children were born. Over the years, of course, babysitters were around too for date nights out, gradually weaving into our lives to become close friends, their children playing with Darcey and Billy like cousins. So the idea of strangers suddenly becoming so intimately involved in our home life was alien to the kids.

Adapting

On top of that, for our children, as for millions of others across the country, lockdown had already changed everything. Months of home learning and then limited interaction, with social distancing, meant that when they were back in school they had been mixing with very few people. The change was destabilising.

For months during lockdown, we had been a tight unit of three. Even when restrictions lifted for others, we still had to be extra-cautious because I couldn't risk infection; otherwise, I would have lost the few hospital visits I was allowed. Home was our sanctuary and in this strange cut-off state I had been able to protect the kids, up to a point, from the full reality of what had happened to their dad. Of course, they were terrified for him and missed him constantly – we couldn't completely escape from reality – but at least I was able to give them some sense of stability.

Dad was in hospital and hospitals made you better – and in the meantime, I, Mum, was here. 'We just have to wait,' I said, and I could see they believed me.

But now there was no hiding the state their dad was in. He was there; they could see the tubes coming out of him that kept him alive; they could see the weakness and they could viscerally feel the tough journey ahead, even if they never doubted that the happy ending we all craved was definitely at the end of it.

What's more, never having been allowed into the hospital, suddenly it must have felt as if the hospital had come to them, into their sanctuary. Not only were there carers in masks and gowns, often two at a time, but there was medical equipment *everywhere!*

Apart from the fact that the sitting room was now Derek's bedroom, with a massive hospital bed in it, there was also a huge mobile hoist to help us get him out of bed. There were special chairs for washing him and transferring him to the wet room, a large extra-supportive wheelchair to transport him, and a specialised separate chair specifically designed to prevent pressure sores and help improve lung function. Unlike the wheelchair (which I now know is miserably uncomfortable and can't have been designed by anyone who has to use one!), the specialised chair allowed us to change his position. This was crucial because we hoped to maximise the time he was out of bed, as his strength increased. We also installed accessibility ramps and a lift to get to the garden.

So, there was no hiding the challenge from Darcey and Billy, or the state their dad was in but, wonderfully, there was no hiding or suppressing the love, either: the flickers of expressions across his face, the affection in his eyes, the moments when love broke through and they could feel his fighting spirit and feed off it. I am so proud of how the kids coped back then and are still coping to this day – their love and spirit spurring me on.

Even when I caught their faces clouding with fear or worry, they would always quickly shake it off, supporting each other with a playful punch or a quick squeeze. 'Don't worry, Bubs,' Darcey would say to Billy. 'It won't be forever – Dad will be fine, you'll see.'

I prayed they were right – firmly pushing away my 'grown-up' fears that the weeks would become months that would turn into years, without any end in sight.

We set up a buzzer on his bed like he'd had in hospital. One of the first things to return as he emerged from the coma and lingered, stuck in a state of minimal consciousness, was the use of his right hand. So we put the buzzer on a string and propped it next to his hand whenever we left the room. It could be heard everywhere in the house: in the kitchen, now our everyday room; just outside the loo; and in my bedroom upstairs. When it went off, it cut through everything: the kids dropped their iPads, and woke up, even from the deepest sleep ... 'Dad, you okay? What do you need?'

He couldn't ask for anything himself, couldn't articulate even the most basic needs – a drink, food, to be warmer, cooler. He was like a baby, only able to cry to show distress or need, so it was a case of running through a checklist: 'Are you cold? Hot? Thirsty?'

He would stare back blankly, but something in his eyes made me think he was struggling to express his thoughts. Or perhaps he was trying to work out the meaning of 'hot' or 'cold' – to make the cogs of his brain move and connect? Sometimes, after what seemed like a lifetime, he'd say, 'Yes, cold,' and I would feel his hands, which were like ice, and wonder how long they had been like that. Twenty minutes later he'd start sweating profusely; his inner thermostat swinging to extremes, his body's weather system out of control, like a jungle in a snowstorm.

He couldn't lie flat for very long and still has to be re-positioned at least once every hour, day and night – any longer and pain creeps in and there is a risk of his muscles and sinews contracting even more. In those early days, we were up all night re-positioning him to try and help him find a moment of relief. Then he would close his eyes, as though just lying still was exhausting, and it was hard to know whether the root of this exhaustion was pain, anxiety or simply the physical effort of keeping his body going.

He was painfully thin. Emaciated. When he first got sick, he lost a devastating amount of weight – eight stone – and when he first came home he started losing masses again, which was terrifying. The hospital had got him to the point of being able to safely chew and swallow tiny amounts of mushed-up food, but it wasn't anywhere near enough to sustain him, let alone increase his strength. It was up to us to ensure that he was hydrated and had all the nutrition he needed, which was hard. We were worried all the time. Very little was known about how Covid affected the gut and the digestive system. Even now the knowledge is piecemeal and anecdotal. But enough people have spoken out about the symptoms to show that it does affect digestion – and Derek was failing to absorb nutrients properly.

We were sustaining him using something called a PEG, a tube that goes into the stomach and extends by about eighteen inches, with a little valve at the end. Food and liquids can go straight in, so we were either puréeing food and putting it into the tube or using a prescription liquid that had all the vitamins and nutrients he needed and was carefully balanced. When making our own puréed food, we had to sterilise all cups or bowls first, by boiling them. The food was administered using a large syringe. Ideally, you would use a new syringe every time, as they do in hospital, but there is no community facility to replace syringes, so I'd boil them, keep them clean and sterilised and replace them regularly.

I remember my hand shaking the first time I sucked up the liquid into the syringe. It seemed like such a terrifying responsibility – literally keeping him alive. You have to make sure there are no air bubbles, sucking up water first to clean the tube and keep it flowing. The liquid food is carefully syringed in, and then you always finish the feed with syringes full of sterile water, to prevent bits of food remaining in any of the tubes, where they could decompose and cause infection. We put the mixture into the PEG at regular intervals throughout the day, trying to keep to a regular pattern, to get Derek's body used to a sense of food going in and going out.

The PEG tube leads to an open hole in the stomach. The skin heals around the tube, but mustn't close tight, because otherwise it could rip. You constantly have to clean it with sterile water; then a piece of foam goes around the hole, sealed with medical tape. We weren't told about the vital step of sealing around it with foam for quite some time, though.

When Derek first came home, we were just cleaning it as best we could. Sometimes the community nurses advised us not to get it wet. 'Keep it dry when you're washing him,' they said. 'Cover it with a plasticised dressing and keep all water away.' Other nurses said that we must wash it and also then wipe around it.

I knew something wasn't right, as he kept getting infections at the PEG site. Then we'd get antibiotics and it would clear up for a while, only to get infected again a few weeks later. I was beginning to learn that, while everyone in the medical profession is extraordinary, some of course have different levels of experience from others. Eventually, a really experienced district nurse visited and said, 'He's getting something called granulation around the PEG site, so you need to put a foam dressing around it to protect it. You need to dress it with the foam protection, then wash it and re-dress it every day.'

It took about two years to get this advice – and in the meantime we were constantly battling infection.

Everything seemed risky. Hydration was an important factor, not only because it's clearly vital for the body to stay hydrated, but also because it eases other challenges like constipation; diet, too, made a huge difference.

As the weeks passed, we urgently needed to weigh Derek. However, there was no scale available in the community that could be used without him standing on it, so he couldn't be weighed. Instead, it was suggested that we measure around his arm to see if he was gaining or losing weight. Although I could see he was losing weight, because he was already so thin, it wasn't particularly visible in his muscles because there was no muscle mass there anyway. Again, it was a case of acting on instinct and trying to convince a nutritionist that even though the measurements of his arm didn't show any particular changes, there was an issue: 'His muscles are so weakened, we can't rely on measuring for the information. We have to get more food into him.'

I talked to everyone I could about the best way to support his nutrition. I read all the information available on the subject and everyone around me chipped in too, desperate to help in any way they could. One day at *GMB,* I realised that the makeup artists and hairdressers, hearing me talking about Derek's nutritional needs on the phone while I was being made up, were doing their own research. They told me to look at an article they'd found and asked what I thought. They'd say 'I heard from a friend of a friend', or they would tell me about something that had made 'all the difference' to someone they knew. They were so loving and supportive.

There were so many questions ... Should he have extra Omega 3 (thought to be good for brain support)? And if so, what was the best way to get that into him? How could we get fibre into a liquid form? Somewhere in among my reading and conversations, I was introduced to moringa, a plant supplement containing proteins, vitamins, minerals and incredible amounts of fibre. In the Indian subcontinent, powdered moringa is often used to combat malnutrition. I mixed it up with water and put it into the feeding tube, and it seemed to inch him forward.

Once he was gaining 'some' weight again, we started thinking about optimising his nutrition. The gut is called the second brain by many scientists and there's lots of research on how your gut health affects your immune system and brain function – some researchers say that what you eat can affect your mood. At least three studies have found that eating more fruits and vegetables is linked with less worry, lower tension and greater life satisfaction, so it made sense to push for the best nutrition to encourage good bacteria in Derek's gut biome, despite the shortcomings of PEG feeding. We had a referral to a community dietician but their ability to help a case like Derek's is limited. Of course, their advice such as 'Eat more fruit and veg' is sound for someone with less damage but we weren't in that position. We needed more specialist nutritionist advice and, despite referrals, we were struggling to get access because knowledge is limited and there are so few experts in this area in the NHS. There are also restrictions as to what they are allowed to recommend: their advice has to be based on decades of confirmed research. The principle of First Do No Harm means that they are very cautious about sanctioning any supplements that might help because they don't yet feel confident enough in the benefits. Like us, the experts are still learning about the true effects of Covid.

Carers who are strangers can't possibly know what would feel normal for Derek, such as how much liquid he usually needs for hydration. I'd had so little time with him while he was in hospital that it felt like the blind leading the blind, yet it's amazing how quickly you learn. We all know water is the elixir of life but as I researched it, I marvelled at just how important it was.

Derek has to have three litres a day – two litres is the normal amount an average person should have in a day, but because of his kidney problems, he needs an additional litre to be flushed through his system. The hospital originally gave us sterile water to hydrate him, but that isn't sustainable in the community, so the nurses advised us to get some large heatproof jugs and fill them up with boiled water, which then had to be allowed to cool. We now make sure that there are always at least three three-litre jugs full of room-temperature water that are constantly replenished.

Liquid intake has to be monitored throughout the day: both liquid in and liquid out. Liquid in is relatively easy to do because we write it down on a piece of paper and the syringe has ml measurements on it, so we just make a note of what goes in. Calculating the liquid out is challenging in somebody who's doubly incontinent, because it involves weighing the pads. We also have to make sure that he isn't retaining liquid in his bladder that could then cause an infection and result in him being sent back to hospital, as has happened several times.

Keeping Derek clean is vital. We have to be scrupulous, always checking, cleaning and swabbing; in every task using the correct monitors, procedures and materials; never cutting corners, always being watchful. I have had to learn a whole new language when it comes to the kit we use. In the early days, we had to get him out of bed to change the sheets sometimes ten times a day, which was a challenge in itself. It took two people. He could begin to reach across his body with one arm; then we would lift him on to his side to change his pad and then roll him back. Sliding sheets allowed us to slide him to one side or the other, but as he couldn't assist, even that simple act took 45 minutes and left us and him exhausted.

At least once a day, we have to get Derek into the wet room, first getting him out of bed and onto a chair with a commode and wheels that can take him into the shower. For this, we have a piece of kit called a Sara Stedy, which looks a bit like a forklift truck with a seat on. Two people are needed to work it: we roll Derek onto his side and, with one person behind, pull him up to a sitting position and move him to the side of the bed. Then, we can both haul him up and quickly release the flap for the seats underneath him, so he's effectively on a high chair on wheels, with his feet on the rolling platform, pitched slightly forward almost as if he's skiing. We wheel it into the wet room and we then have to repeat the procedure to get him to the kit that keeps him safe in the shower – and then wash him and do everything again in reverse. Initially, it could sometimes take an hour or more, and then he'd need a wash.

Things can go wrong at any time, as I was reminded on Bonfire Night in 2021. The kids were out at their school fireworks display and I was at home caring for Derek, along with a female carer. The carer and I were lifting him from the bed to take him to the wet room, because he needed to be washed; as we got him up, we slightly mistimed placing his feet on the Sara Stedy. He went down and as he did, I quickly put my body underneath his bottom to prevent him hitting the ground. But then we were stuck there; unable to get Derek up, and only just preventing him from falling further ... But for how long could we hold him? My back felt as if it was breaking, and I could see the carer sweating with fear.

She couldn't get him up. I called for Tommy, our babysitter, who was there as well, so that while I was dealing with Derek she could look after the children when they got back. She's really strong, and plays a lot of football, but even the three of us, with me pushing from underneath, couldn't lift him the few inches needed to get him back up onto the Sara Stedy, where his bottom is perched when he's being moved.

In the weeks leading up to this moment, Derek had started getting much stronger and it had been much easier to feel confident that we could do this. But his fatigue is so unpredictable. It can just shut him down at any point – a bit like a computer crashing – and when it strikes, it's as if he's been drugged. His muscles are like jelly and he has no control, so he's a dead weight.

For about an hour, we tried to lift him. He said he wasn't in pain but was obviously very distressed – as we were – and we were also worried because we didn't want him to fall down any further. If that happened, I knew we definitely wouldn't get him back up. Also, I didn't want his full weight to go down onto his buckled legs as they were so stick-thin, I feared they might end up breaking.

Billy came home ahead of Darcey. As he came in the door, I shouted through the hall, 'Billy, come in here!'

'Oh my God!' Billy said, seeing this extraordinary tableau.

I told Billy to go and get our neighbour, Simon, as I wanted to see if a fourth pair of hands could help to lift Derek. By this point, I'd been supporting Derek's weight on my hands and knees in a cat position, with Tommy and the carer helping from above. My whole body was shaking from the strain and I'm sure they were struggling too.

Billy came back without Simon and shouted, 'He's not there! He's at the fireworks!'

Darcey then got home with a friend, Polly, and her parents, who had walked them back to the house. 'Darcey,' I said, 'quickly run back out and grab Polly's parents before they go – and ask if Polly's dad can come and help.'

I was aware that this was a really humiliating and scary situation for Derek, so when I heard Polly's dad coming, I said, 'Are you okay with them coming in, bearing in mind you've never met Polly's dad?'

At that point, he came out with one of the first long sentences he'd uttered since he came out of his coma: 'I'm aware of the predicament I'm in, Kate. Yes, of course, you must get help.'

It was a really strange moment, one of total fear and total wonder. 'Oh my God, he's Derek, he is in there – he gets it!' as well as 'Oh my God, he couldn't be more vulnerable at this point.'

But there was no time to dwell on that.

I looked up, and turned to Polly's dad. 'Listen, I'm so sorry. We've never met ...'

He was absolutely lovely. 'Ah, Derek Draper, it's good to meet you. I've heard lots about you from Polly. Let's see if we can get this sorted out.'

Thankfully, with Polly's dad's extra muscle and Darcey

helping too, the five of us heaved him up just enough to get him back on the Sara Stedy and then get him back into bed. It was a huge reminder of how quickly things can escalate and even with the carers there 24 hours a day, we could never be totally sure that things wouldn't go wrong.

It was also a reminder of the kindness of people in moments of crisis and I like to remember this because when you are caring for someone you tend to just move on to the next challenge and, if you don't hold on to those positive moments, they can get lost. There's always uncertainty, and scary moments come up when you least expect them, but so do the lovely ones too.

At first, we were often in a fug of tiredness, especially Derek, whose every movement rendered him exhausted, as though he had just run a marathon. But amid the exhaustion came moments of tenderness and love. Remember, Derek is very sensitive to touch, as if it burns him or triggers too much sensation. The shower we'd installed was overwhelming – he recoiled at the feeling of water beating down on his body. He'd always been a bath person before and now I worried that with his new skin sensitivity we were almost torturing him. I could only imagine how it must have felt after more than a year of having bed baths. But as I stroked him, trying to gently cleanse and introduce the shower, I saw trust in his eyes, a loving look; I saw him mouth 'Thank you.'

Adapting

How long had it been since I'd smoothed my fingers across his skin? Physical love felt so natural, so beautiful, in these moments. We were making contact elementally, speaking our own language, communicating without words, as lovers do. And these were some of the moments, however fleeting, that kept me going as my world revolved around Derek's recovery.

On the other hand, I've often been at the less fragrant end of caring, dealing with poo – yet, even then, Derek and I have experienced the most intense moments of shared love. After one poo episode (and there have been many), I said to him – on my knees on the floor with a bucket, sponging it up – 'When we stood on the steps of St Mary's Church on our first date, and then again, a year later, on our wedding day, I don't remember this ever being mentioned as a possible future scenario.'

He laughed and then cried and mouthed 'Love you'; and then a pause and with a deeply tender look in his eye: 'Sorry.'

I was in awe of his ability to fight on, despite the obstacles, and that gave me the strength to fight on *for* him. I put that strength down to love, which gives you the power to take on what you never thought possible, things you couldn't have done to or for a stranger. It overrides anxiety and – especially when I was desperately wishing I had some medical training or at least a bit of previous experience of doing what I was doing – it was my companion and guide. Loving someone means caring that much more, which gives you strength to lift when you don't believe you can. And it keeps you going when you're dead on your feet and every muscle aches to the point of shaking.

These moments reminded me that Derek was at home not only because we loved him and wanted him to be there, it was for his own good. Being at home gave him more chance of getting better; we were part of his recovery, wrapping our love around him, giving him the motivation to push forward and recover.

Chapter 5

Who Cares About Care?

Care – the actual act of caring for someone – never gets the credit it deserves, does it? I don't just mean in terms of wages for professional carers and recognition of the vital role they play in our society (which in my view should definetely be more in both cases, but here is not the place to tackle that). No, I'm talking in terms of perception – the glamour, the importance, the sexiness and the veneration that other areas of the medical profession seem to attract and that caring, whether it's done for money or love, just doesn't.

Think of the dramas you see on TV and at the movies. In about five seconds, I can count dozens based around accident and emergency departments and hospitals generally. The drama of watching people save lives never loses its appeal – it's always a ratings winner, forever fascinating, and that fascination with life-saving engages us with the characters as people, too. We are intrigued by their personalities, by what drives and motivates them, and how they attempt to weave their demanding jobs into lives that swirl with all the normal desires and challenges, such as friendships, family, love and ambition. Admittedly, these characters are much easier to hook onto when they are played by the likes of George Clooney, *ER*'s heartthrob paediatrician (I have interviewed him several times and, believe me, he could stand in front of a wall watching paint dry and we'd still all queue up for tickets to see!); or Sandra Oh, as the ultra-competitive surgeon in *Grey's Anatomy* – and not forgetting Hugh Laurie's flawed clinician in *House* and, of course, countless others.

But I've yet to see such a show based around the slow meticulous work of carers, even though caring involves just as much minute-by-minute tension, while their lives are every bit as challenging and complex. Why is that? Is it simply that we have all experienced in some way the drama of the hospital? Is it fear that drives us to make sense of it, to know more about the people who inhabit that scary world and then, in that comforting way that TV and films do, have everything wrapped up by the end so we can feel reassured?

When we enter a hospital we see glimpses of crisis all around us: the pinched face of an anxious relative, hands clasped, waiting for news; the quiet rush of air as a nurse in scrubs hurries past; the bandaged schoolboy on crutches, limping out of the lift with his mum; the frail old lady half-asleep on a trolley parked outside a ward; the expectant mother tentatively lumbering towards the maternity unit. And somewhere at the centre of things, we sense, is a mysterious portal with two doors, one leading out into the sunshine and the other … elsewhere. It's no surprise that we're fascinated by the highly skilled doctors and nurses we see in action in hospitals, even if just fleetingly, and that watching their god-like powers as they battle to save our lives makes us wonder, *Who are these people?*

But have you ever wondered who a carer is? What are *their* dreams? How did *they* come to be doing what they are doing? It certainly seems Hollywood doesn't.

Why is that? Is it our lack of curiosity? Is it because the work of caring is subtler, less visible and in fact represents a part of our life that we don't want to think about until it's right there in our face? Or is it because the length of time it usually takes for the benefits of caring to unfold isn't an easy fit for an hour-long episode? As I now live the life of a carer and see professional carers at work, I know that it's no less full of jeopardy and that it's just as relentlessly stressful as the work in any busy hospital ward, but it isn't perceived as 'high stakes', even though lives are just as dependent on it. Caring is for the long haul, an ongoing process of nudging somebody towards recovery, or sometimes just struggling to maintain the status quo. The remit isn't always clear-cut – there may be no real sense of where it's going to lead or if you're going to get the result you want. Hospital treatment is more easily defined: it can feel very black and white – recover or don't, live or die – while caring is more about the grey area in between.

While it's not as obvious, believe me there's no less jeopardy or healing power in caring. In fact, it is the very essence of all healing. It's just that we don't recognise the drama and the power of it. I learned the power of care in one of the most dramatic moments in our journey with Derek – and, ironically, I learned it from a *hospital* doctor.

At this point, the first hospital Derek had been admitted to was struggling to save his life and the doctors knew they were losing the battle; the leader of the unit called me to relate the grim news. The only hope was a transfer to another hospital, where they had a piece of kit that might buy him more time for his body to fight the infection. This was the ECMO machine which I have previously described. We had no idea when his name would come up for transfer, or if it would be in time. Then I suddenly got the call – the team were on their way to move him. Relief. But when they arrived, there was another call, not to say he was on his way, but that he was too sick to be moved. He wouldn't survive the journey, they said. It was impossible.

'But it can't be impossible, can it? There must be something you can try?' I insisted.

Doing nothing and letting him slip away was *not* an option. I couldn't let it be; I was running on adrenaline like the people in those TV shows; I wanted George Clooney to be there shouting, 'Get a major haemorrhage pack, stat!' as he raced to grab another piece of kit, or Hugh Laurie from *House* asking the crucial question that made the unexplainable explainable, the impossible possible.

There was an option, the doctor said, but it wasn't a good one: taking him to surgery there, in that hospital, and inserting the necessary tubes to start him on ECMO *before* the transfer. But he was so weak, it was high-risk – he might die.

'Can you do that, then?' I pushed.

'We can try, but it won't be easy or quick. Because of the Covid restrictions it takes 14 hours to sanitise the theatre between operations and staff numbers are very restricted, too.'

I resisted thinking too much about all these barriers, focusing instead on the hope and the light of the one option that might save him.

'Can we try?'

'I'll get back to you.'

Half an hour later. 'Good news,' the team leader said. 'Because of Covid the hospital is overwhelmed so there are no operations booked; other patients aren't suitable for ECMO and one theatre is free.'

It's hard to remember how hard those times were and to think about a situation where a hospital *overwhelmed* with hundreds of people fighting for their lives from an untreatable and potentially fatal virus could be good news for anyone. But at that point, for Derek, it was. I felt guilty, but also so grateful. 'Sending love to all those others and their terrified relatives, God bless you,' I said in my head.

The team leader's voice brought me back to Derek.

'A surgeon is getting ready and putting on the PPE so we *can* try, but I need to be sure you know the risks in case, in case ...' he faltered.

'In case something goes wrong and I blame you?' I finished.

'Well, I wouldn't have put it as bluntly as that, but essentially yes.'

As Derek was in a deep coma, I had to run through a next-of-kin checklist and decide whether or not we should go ahead. It was a terrifying responsibility, but what choice did I have?

I answered the questions as best I could, confirming that I knew all the risks: heart failure, stroke, seizures, lung collapse, multiple blood loss – the potential horrors went on and on. And at the end I had one question for the doctor: 'What will happen if we *don't* do this?'

Long pause on the other end of the line.

'Well, we can never really know, because the human body has a way of surprising even the best doctors,' he said eventually. 'But looking at him now, I have to say that in my opinion he will certainly die.'

'Then there doesn't really seem to be a choice, does there? We can't just give up. We have to fight to give him the best chance we can.'

'Okay, we'll do it,' he said, adding, 'Don't worry, we will take good care of him.'

He said this in that casual way we all do. For instance, when someone says in a restaurant, 'Could you keep an eye on my handbag while I go to the loo?' you reply, 'Sure, I'll take care of it.' The implication is 'That won't be a problem; I'll make sure nothing happens to it,' and in your head you think, *It's not going to trouble me beyond giving it a cursory glance now and then.*

However, I knew 'take care of' in this case meant something very different, something much more vital which would require huge effort and skill, despite the relaxed way it was communicated.

They rushed him into theatre to insert the tubes, which was not an easy procedure. Later I found out that while I'd been waiting for news with my heart in my mouth, Derek's heart had stopped altogether. Mercifully, they got it going again within seconds. It highlighted how much they had to take 'care' during the procedure.

Then began the agonising journey across London, going impossibly slowly, because every jolt might dislodge a vital tube. Yet not too slowly, because they knew that every second lost increased the risk of him not making it there alive. The team promised to call as soon as the ambulance arrived at the new hospital.

We were still at the height of Covid, when no one could visit, and I agonised about what might be happening as the minutes turned into hours. I pictured the team meticulously checking every monitor, every beep, making sure they did everything they could to help him survive the journey, knowing that this care was the only thing keeping him alive. Derek knew nothing of any of this, of course – he was still in the coma – nothing of the strangers holding his life by the thinnest of threads, nor that their 'care' was giving this thread the strength of reinforced steel and that without it, it would have snapped like a strand of cotton. It was a comfort to me, though, that he was not aware of the jeopardy and not in pain.

Having given the kids the barest details about what was happening, I tried to play a game with them to distract myself. But every time the phone flashed with a message I ran to it, hoping it was the ambulance team.

It was nearly midnight before they called.

'Did he make it?' I burst out, before the doctor had even had a chance to properly introduce himself.

'Yes, he made it. But ...'

Oh, I hated those buts.

'Look, the only way I can say this is he's very, very ill and he really might not pull through. We have got him here, but it's still precarious. Now we need to scan him from top to toe and get some medicines into him. I'll know more in the morning. Try to get some sleep.'

Sleep didn't come easily, as you can imagine, but the idea of 'getting medicines into him' sounded promising. Something concrete, something proactive that might actually help. Something other than 'wait and see'. We have been programmed since we were kids, haven't we, that medicines are the answer? The doctor will give you some pills or a spoonful of something and that will make you better.

It was nearly lunchtime the following day before the doctor called back.

'Is he alive?' As always, this was my first question.

'Yes, he's still alive, and the ECMO seems to be functioning well, but ...'

Again, the dreaded 'but'.

'... we'll just have to see how the next few hours and the next couple of days go.'

'I see,' I said, trying to take in what he really meant, not wanting to let him off the phone until he gave me something more tangible, a shred of hope to stabilise my mind during the agony of waiting.

'And what about getting the medicines into him – when can you start doing that?'

'Medicines? What do you mean, medicines?' asked the voice on the other end of the phone.

'You said last night you wanted to get some medicines into him and then see how things were.'

'Oh, I'm sorry. I think you misunderstood me. There are no medicines for Covid. Nothing can cure it.'

'No, I know that. So, hang on, what medicines did you mean, then?'

Remember, this was 2020, when the global biotech community were frantically investigating antibodies and scrabbling to find existing drugs that might be effectively repurposed for Covid, when vaccines were still so far from being developed that they were almost a pipe dream.

'Well, there are drugs we can use to stabilise the heart and to keep the kidneys working better on the dialysis, and drugs to help the blood flow more easily so the ECMO has a chance to do its job. We have to balance the amount of blood thinners we put in to keep the blood moving; we know now that Covid makes the blood sticky, so we have to keep it moving around the body to keep the oxygen going to all the vital organs. But we have to balance that against the risk of bleeding, either at the site where the tubes go in – he had a big bleed there overnight, by the way – or elsewhere like, God forbid, on the brain.'

'Right,' I said slowly, trying to piece together what all this meant for Derek right here, right now. 'So you can't actually *do* anything to make him better? It's nothing but wait and see. Where is the hope going to come from?'

I was trying to process my thoughts, barely realising I was expressing them audibly, and I wish I hadn't said what I was thinking out loud, because it must have sounded so rude.

'Well, I wouldn't say what we are doing is *nothing!*' he bridled.

'God, no, sorry, I didn't mean it like that – of course you are doing *everything!* You are keeping him alive. I just meant – what next? What is going to turn this around? What will bring him back to us, other than prayers and letting Covid take its course?'

He was quiet for a very long time. I began to wonder if I had offended him so much that he had hung up.

Then I heard him take a deep breath.

'Very, very good *care*. That's what is going to save him. Incredible care is our weapon in this war. It's the weapon in every medical war, really.'

Now I was the one who fell silent. I felt winded. Care? Only care?! The word seemed so lightweight, so flimsy, so ineffectual in fighting the savageness of this disease. I imagined a concerned nurse mopping Derek's brow with a gloved hand, checking her fob watch, like Florence Nightingale, and taking his pulse, tutting, noting it down and walking to the next patient to do the same.

As if he had read my mind, the doctor continued, 'People think care is just brow mopping and bottom wiping, but care is actually the basis of all medicine. It's observation, which informs decision-making, it's the critical action of noticing and reacting accordingly, of paying attention to every detail and extrapolating what might be important and focusing on it. It's the fundamental of medicine, the humanity that transforms medical practice from a bunch of chemicals in a pharmacy, or a diagram in a textbook, to life-saving action. The best medicine is very good care.

'We constantly monitor blood pressure and heart rate, adjust the medication to stabilise and press in the right direction, note and adjust oxygen levels, push what will work, note down what doesn't. We are doing everything to sustain him; it's the care that will give him his best chance of surviving.

'*Good care* is certainly not *nothing*.'

Crikey, it was a lot to take in. I'd clearly struck a nerve with this doctor. And today this point totally strikes a chord with me. I now know that care is life-saving, it *is* life and death and just as dramatically vital as the work of the wonderful medical teams in a hospital.

* * *

Derek was home now – and very, very good care was our best hope of him surviving and progressing. And as the weeks turned into months, and then into years, I would truly *feel* what that doctor had meant. I would truly *live* that care isn't nothing. It is, in fact, *everything*.

I learned that even the seemingly 'simplest' of care tasks was fraught with medical complexity, just as that doctor had described. Take the straightforward instruction 'Keep patient hydrated.' Even the most inexperienced carer would know that means 'make sure the patient has enough water', but how much is enough and what is the impact of having too much or too little?

What does water really do for us?

As I soon discovered, asking *that* question is a bit like when Reg in *The Life of Brian* asks his People's Front of Judea mates, 'What have the Romans ever done for us?', hoping to prove they have done nothing and deserve to be overthrown. Instead, he gets a whole stream of answers that show the Romans have changed their world for the better. And, as I soon found out, the joke is even more apt when querying the importance of water because, while the Romans could be a huge civilising force, water is the source of all life, the essence of existence, the one substance NASA scientists search for on alien planets to see if there's a chance that living things have ever, or could ever, thrive amid their boiling lava and frozen atmospheres. And it makes up at least half of our human bodies.

Wait, I'm only just getting started ...

Now that I knew the *value* of care, it meant steeping myself in new information about everything – and even just the facts I discovered about water are mind-blowing.

Let's start with the skin, our largest organ, which is made up of 20 per cent water. When your skin loses moisture, this level can drop to below 10 per cent, affecting your level of collagen, which gives your skin elasticity and keeps it firm. Dehydration causes wrinkles, so you should drink more water to stay looking younger – you've heard that before, I'm sure. But don't think those shrivelling concerns are only skin-deep, because that 'wrinkling' is going on inside, too, in every other organ in your body.

When dehydrated, the liver's function decreases because it no longer has sufficient water to help flush out waste. Derek's liver had been in crisis and its long-term functioning was still unknown so keeping hydrated was vital for this, as well as for the health of his other organs. As water makes up most of your blood, too, hydration makes it easier for your blood to pass through the liver and be filtered. Basically, the less hydrated you are, the less efficient your liver is at filtering out toxins.

We could see with our own eyes that breathing was a desperate struggle for Derek and that administering the right amount of water could perhaps ease this for him a little. Drinking water helps to thin the mucus lining in your airways and lungs – lack of moisture can cause that mucus to gunk up, slowing down overall respiration and in turn making you more susceptible to infection, allergies and other breathing problems. It makes the struggle of breathing in and out harder, and also contributes to a depleted amount of oxygen passing through the tubes of the lungs to the blood.

Covid had left Derek with two holes in his heart and vast swings in blood pressure, plummeting from terrifyingly high to dangerously low. Dehydration leads to a decrease in blood volume, as water is lost from the body, and this reduction in blood volume means there is less fluid available for the heart to pump. As a result, the heart has to work harder to maintain an adequate blood flow around the body, leading to an increase in heart rate, which can be an additional strain.

Blood pressure changes when you're dehydrated because a rise in sodium levels triggers the release of a hormone called vasopressin, which works to help your body retain water. Then, because the blood vessels (arteries, capillaries, veins and others) need water to stay 'full', vasopressin squeezes them to make them smaller and keep them flowing. This tightening in the vessels leads to higher blood pressure and suddenly you are heading towards heart attack, embolism and stroke territory. Severe dehydration can also cause your blood volume to decrease, which in turn can cause a blood pressure *drop*, leading to lightheadedness, dizziness, and potential fainting episodes.

Derek had suffered all these symptoms at various points and continues to. So making sure he was hydrated was even more important. He'd also endured acute kidney failure twice and been on dialysis for months; his kidneys required constant scrutiny. The degree to which the function was impaired was still unknown, but doctors told us it was likely to be poor, as dehydration impairs the kidneys' ability to get rid of waste, which means you have toxins hanging around – never a good idea – and it prompts the kidneys to try and conserve water by producing less urine. Darker, more concentrated urine potentially irritates the bladder lining and increases the risk of urinary tract infections, which he was already prone to. Even worse, the minerals and salts in concentrated urine can crystallise, clump together and start forming kidney stones, as Derek discovered with near-fatal consequences when, a year after he'd come home, he had to go back into hospital having developed sepsis from kidney stones and kidney malfunction, which threatened his life all over again.

Water is so important for the brain, too. It clears out the toxins and waste that impair brain function and also carries nutrients to your brain to keep it healthy. It helps your brain cells communicate with each other, which is vital for even the most basic thinking and brain–body connection. It is also crucial for everyday functioning: staying hydrated has been linked to better concentration, focus, short-term memory, learning ability, cognitive functioning, mental energy and alertness.

If you become dehydrated, a lot of these positives are reversed and, what's more, you can become irritable and indecisive, get a headache, start feeling unsure of yourself and even physically unbalanced. There are some studies that also suggest lack of water can compound depression. We knew Derek had difficulty with trying to focus, with slow processing and poor memory; also with retrieving information from his brain and finding a way to link that with his mouth in order to communicate. We knew his cognition and communication were incredibly impaired. It was unlikely that all this was just down to dehydration, but we were learning that the effects of damage from Covid to his brain and nervous system were only going to be made worse by a lack of water.

Becoming dehydrated can even be life-threatening; it can cause seizures, brain inflammation, kidney failure; it can put you into shock or a coma, and possibly kill you. Sobering, isn't it? And all this just from a lack of an appropriate amount of water. That simple, colourless, tasteless stuff that flows out of the tap.

And 'appropriate' is the key word here, because consuming too much water can also have disastrous consequences. Known as water intoxication or water poisoning, over-hydration can, in severe cases, be fatal. So, too much leads to disaster, and so does too little, revealing the perils of just this one apparently simple care task of 'Keep patient hydrated.'

For most people, the body has clever ways to prevent too much or too little hydration. Thirst is a key one, signalling we need to drink, and a sense of nausea being another, when we've had too much. But of course, Derek couldn't recognise thirst. He didn't seem to have any sense of dehydration and couldn't express it either, so too much or too little was a high risk.

And of course, hydration wasn't our only care challenge. The carers and I now faced dozens and dozens – hundreds, even – of priorities like this, with similar precarious balances. From administering his medication, to his skin and his movement, from his muscles to his bones, his digestive system and secretions, his ability to focus and communicate ...

I won't list them all – and all their consequences – because it would take forever, but I think you get the drift! It was akin to walking a tightrope, knowing that the smallest slip could put Derek at risk. And yet, when done properly, care is life-saving and life-giving.

Now I truly 'got' what that doctor meant. Every minute we were checking, re-checking, weighing, measuring, moving, cleaning, monitoring and observing: the careful observation of the flicker of an eye, the change in colour of complexion or an unexpected wince – all these signs gave us valuable information about what was happening with Derek. He was our project and, almost without realising, the kids and I were consciously observing his every move. Any tiny change was vital information for the experts and had to be passed on to the next carer who arrived, just as they passed on information to us.

I was proud of how the kids were coping with all this. But I also worried about what effect it might be having on them. Was it adding to their stress levels? All this precision and focus on sickness every day, when they should be left to be children, to grow and be carefree? And indeed, what effect was it having on Derek himself? Were we adding to the pressure on him, by – in a sense – caring *too much*? Was it creating more anxiety for everyone? In fact, it seemed to help, and in the most extraordinary way.

I've talked already about how needing to be constantly alive to Derek's needs, and for months not knowing whether he would live or die, had placed us in a constant state of adrenaline-fuelled, flight-or-fight anxiety. That was why I worried that caring for Derek in this way might actually be making things worse. But, having read extensively about the human brain in an effort to understand what Covid had done to Derek's brain, and how best to *care* for him, I began to see how to manage this constant pressure.

The human brain has one purpose – as an incredibly effective survival machine, which can work for us or against us, depending what we program into it. Picture our ancestors, always on the lookout for predators, scarce resources or hazards. It was crucial for them to stay alert and react swiftly, and their brains delivered. This mindset, known as the 'negativity bias', has been hardwired into our brains through natural selection, because only those who spotted threats and reacted to them survived. As a result of this hardwiring, thousands of generations later, negative or threatening information still grabs our attention more intensely than positive or neutral information. That's why the most shocking news headlines are the ones that get our attention. It's our brains saying, 'Hey, pay attention – potential risk for you. Check this out!'

On top of that, our memory is like a giant library that supports the brain. When we are in trouble, our brain scans our memories to look for ways to avoid a threat. It's why we often remember the bad things more than the good things. It's not that humans are simply negative, it's just that our brain's priority is risk, not whether we are happy.

When I was little, like many kids, I used to love 'doing a Peppa Pig', jumping in muddy puddles; I remember walking to the shop with my mum, revelling in the big splashes I created along the way. And then one day I jumped in a puddle that was deeper; it had a hole hidden beneath its flat, still surface and so when I jumped, the water came over the top of my wellies. Shock! I then had a long walk home with cold, wet feet and sopping socks that rubbed against my boots.

The next time I went out with my parents, I still wanted to jump, but I remembered what had happened. And my brain, almost without my being aware of it, had learned to assess what a deep, welly-flooding puddle looked like. I don't know if it was something about the reflection of the light on the water or the ripples on the surface, and I didn't have to know, as my brain had done the work for me. It had connected the dots of my *feelings*, the shock and the discomfort of my feet, and used the data from my eyes to protect me from this potential risk. Clever, huh?

This is also of course why we have to pay attention to the feelings we are feeding into our supercomputer brains, because if we think negatively our brains will sense danger. And the brain doesn't unpick the danger – that's our job – it just focuses on our need to survive.

In fact I still jumped in muddy puddles, probably thanks to my parents saying, 'Go on, don't be afraid: have fun!', so their positive enthusiasm offset the fear and my brain did the rest. I never had such a soaking again, at least not until I was older and there was alcohol involved!

However, this survival mechanism – the brain being constantly alert to keep us safe – can also lead to stress and random anxiety. We have to find a way of consciously teaching our brain that a particular danger isn't a priority; that we don't need to worry about it right then. A sabre-toothed tiger at the door of the cave? Definitely a problem, because in Neanderthal times (no ambulances, no pain-killers), it was vital to be alert to predators. But in modern times, our adrenaline gets released even when something isn't an immediate danger – and we don't know what to do with it.

For example, if there's a car crash right in front of you while you're driving, your brain instinctively and quite rightly responds to the immediate threat to keep you safe. However, if you hear about a crash some-where not in your immediate vicinity, your brain might at first jump into survival mode – thinking about what caused the crash, and whether the same thing might happen to you – and it's up to you to then ascertain whether there is in fact any real danger to you. And if you manage to do that, you will begin to calm the fight/flight response.

Historically, our brain used our senses to ascertain threat. Today, though, the presence of 24-hour news bulletins and social media brings threat immediately into our everyday lives, even though what we are consuming might not present a real risk to us. It is up to us to process the information for our brain and to work out what, if any, danger there really is. In recent years in particular, there has been so much negative information flying at us that our brains are reeling, leaving us with a sense of anxiety. Our brains can't turn off that survival instinct, so they run away with us, because we are powerless to resolve the fear.

Our brains hate this powerlessness. This is why having a plan is so helpful. The brain thrives on structure and control. When you have a clear goal and a plan to achieve it, you're giving your brain something to focus on. It's like saying, 'Hey, brain, instead of worrying about the random things that you can't control, concentrate on this specific task instead.' And so the focus and the precision of caring for Derek was giving our family a plan, a roadmap to help deal with the uncertainty of his health. Wonderfully, this gave me an even stronger bond with Derek, fostering his trust in me and connecting us on a primeval level of survival.

Caring for Derek in this way also sparked a new sense of wonder in me about the human body and gave me a greater understanding of how all our organs interconnect. When you think of how simple tasks not done in the right way can lead to such catastrophic results, it's a miracle that things don't go wrong more often. And my awe wasn't only reserved for the human body, but also for the human spirit, for Derek's spirit that made him plough on, fight for life and seize it, and for the extraordinary spirit of carers everywhere who support that fight for life.

It seemed to bring wonder into the kids' lives too. They marvelled at all the new things we were learning. I talked to them about how we could use the knowledge to bolster our own health. It was as though Derek, by accident, was teaching us the importance of self-care.

When they heard me talking about giving water to Derek and discussing the importance of correct hydration with the carers, they started asking me questions about it. They were fascinated. They started drinking more themselves. Billy had been having a lot of headaches and tummy aches – probably partly due to stress, or at least worry certainly didn't help – along with disrupted sleep, but when he heard how water was important to help 'Daddy's head', he asked me if drinking more water would help him as well; I said yes and he started to do it. And it *did* help. Yes, water really does aid digestion; it improves sleep, too, and eases headaches. But it also helped him mentally: got him thinking about the fact that he had some control over his body, maybe even over his painful feelings. I could see the beneficial effects on him and realised that this was a positive in a sea of negatives. Caring for Derek and learning about what his new needs were was teaching Billy how to be physically stronger and more self-reliant, giving him confidence that he could make things better for himself, physically and mentally.

As I thought about this, I felt a stab of guilt. Was it bad to feel anything but horror at this awful situation Derek was in? Was it wrong to see any 'positive'? I understood we had to find joy *along* the way to keep the kids and I sane, but this was different. This was a positive thought *because* of the horror, not *in spite* of it. When I looked at Derek's wracked body and thought of his imprisoned mind, it felt deeply wrong to my core to think that anything good could come out of this. That's what the insidious emotion guilt does – it destroys gratitude and attacks the vital need for a positive outlook to get you through any crisis.

But, for now, it was Derek himself who showed me how to see this positive in the best light. One day he was really struggling. I now knew how to look for the signs and I could see he was dehydrated, so I said, 'Let's get some more water into you.'

I prepared some cooled, boiled water, sterilised the syringes and began to feed water through his PEG – the tube going into his stomach that keeps him alive with liquid 'food' and vital hydration.

Billy was sitting there fascinated, mesmerised. Derek looked at him and then looked back at me with tears in his eyes.

'Oh God, does he hate the idea of Billy watching?' I thought. 'Does he not want him to see something so intimate? Maybe he doesn't like being so vulnerable in front of his son. Although it had never worried him before.'

'Is it bothering you that Billy is watching?' I asked.

He nodded.

In a way, this was a moment in itself. The fact that he had been able to recognise and express the emotion of feeling uncomfortable with a situation, rather than just the smiles and looks of love which, although wonderful, were much more simplistic. This felt more complex, more like he was in touch with himself; it felt like progress, albeit in a tragic way.

'Don't worry, Dad,' said Billy, 'I'll go.'

'No, don't go,' Derek whispered, then looked at me and said, 'Shame.'

'What's a shame?' Billy asked.

But I knew it was a different type of shame.

'You feel ashamed?' I asked.

A tiny nod.

'Why? You have nothing to feel ashamed about,' I said.

Derek looked at Billy and whispered, 'I have let you down. I can't be your dad.'

Billy's eyes widened. 'Don't be silly, Dad, you haven't let me down. You are my hero. You are so brave; you're amazing – you're Indiana Jones and Luke Skywalker, with a bit of Han Solo thrown in.'

Derek smiled and sobbed. Billy was over-egging it with his favourite screen heroes, but it was working.

I knew, though, what Derek was feeling: that he couldn't do anything and was too weak even to move towards Billy for a hug. He had been the person who taught Billy to walk, to talk, to drink from a sippy cup and then a grown-up cup. Now, here he was, unable to even take a sip for himself, relying on others to get water into his body.

'I just want to be your dad again,' Derek mouthed. There was no 'note' to his voice, no vibration of the vocal cords to make a sound. He mouthed the words and the air came so strongly we could hear, *feel,* it come from deep within him.

'Oh Dad!' Billy's voice was full of emotion too.

He craned forward to half-lie next to Derek and hug him, careful not to crush or hurt him. Derek continued to sob.

I waited, letting them hold each other, hold each other's emotions and fears. Father and son.

Then, sensing that neither knew how to break this – to stop – I ventured, 'Derek, you might think you're not being a dad, but us taking care of you is teaching Billy. He now drinks loads of water – so you are still teaching him, still parenting him.'

'Yes, Dad, *you* did that!' said Billy – God bless him for getting it.

'Still your dad, love you, love you,' Derek mumbled over and over again, through muffled sobs.

'Yes, Dad, and you always will be,' said Billy, 'and also this ... this,' he searched for the word, '*state* you are in won't be forever. You *will* get better. We have a plan. We can do it together.'

Yes, we had a plan: we just had to keep going. We had love and care – and what is caring for someone, other than an act of love? And in that moment, I believed that Billy was right. If the strength of our love was anything to go by, somehow we truly could.

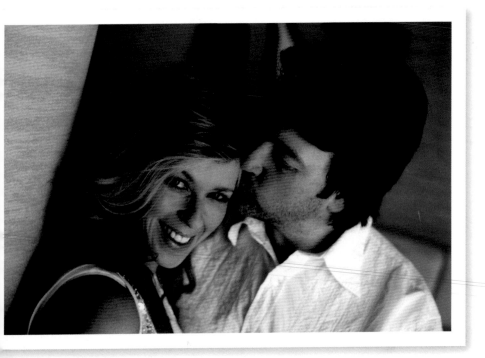

In Derek's wedding speech he vowed to care for me through life's ups and downs.

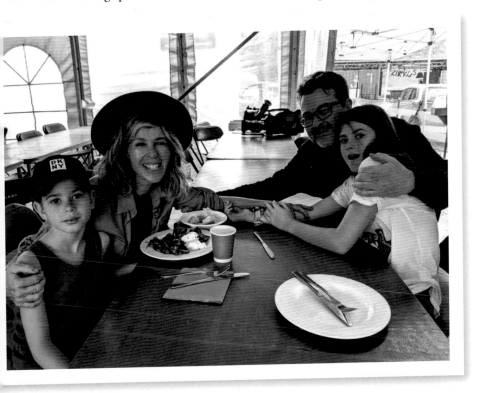

Reunited with the family after leaving the *I'm A Celebrity* … jungle –
proper food at last!

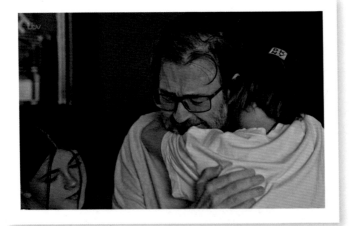

Left: Home at last – the emotional momen when Derek and the kids saw each other again for the first tim

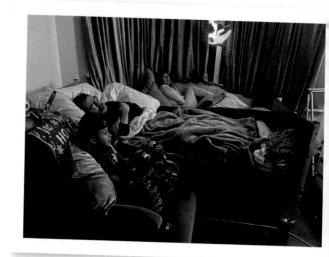

Right: The Christmas we feared we'd never share as a family. Christmas Day 2021.

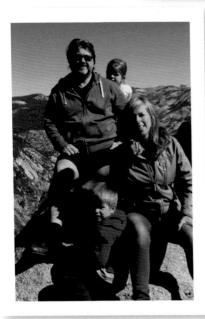

Left: One of Derek's amazing family adventures. On this trip, we visited some of America's incredible national parks.

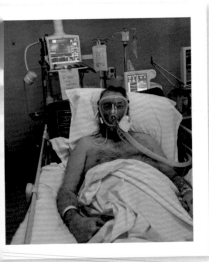

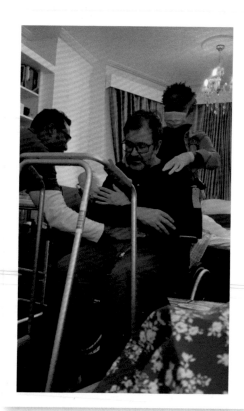

Derek spent months in a coma and more than a year in the clinical hospital environment. Even in a sitting position, he needs two people to stabilise him … so it was a huge moment when he was strong enough to come into the garden to reconnect with nature.

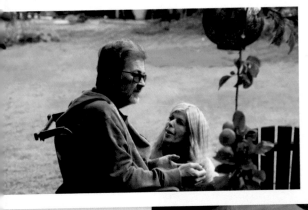

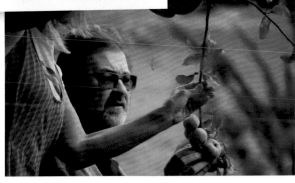

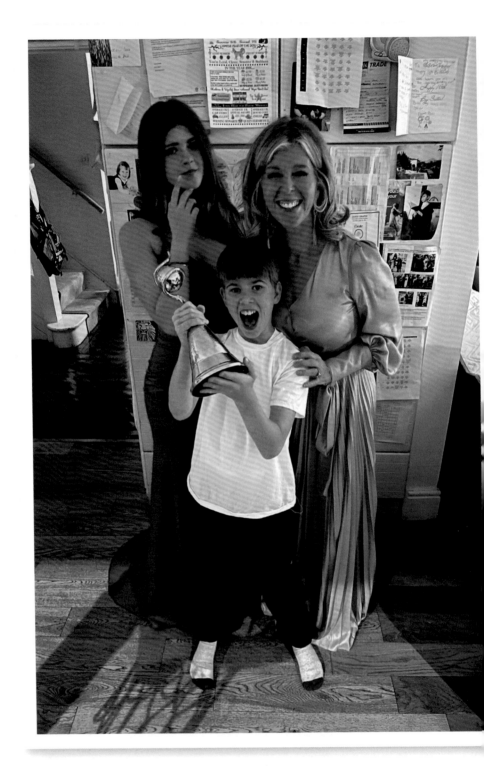

Darcey and Bill were so proud and excited when Derek and I won the National Television Awards for our documentaries *Finding Derek* and *Caring for Derek*. Pictur[e] behind us is the fridge door that mustn't be rearranged!

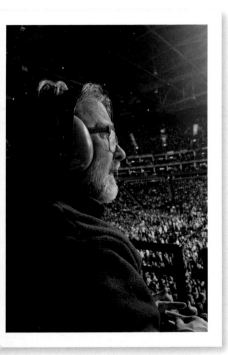
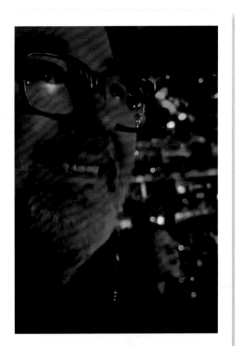
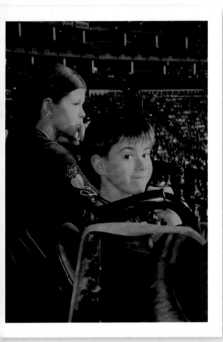
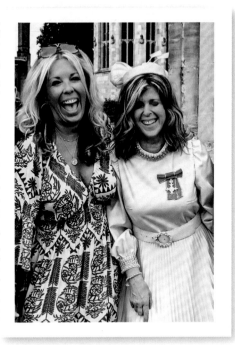

Top and below left: What a night! Sir Elton John's music has been so powerful in helping Derek throughout all of this and he has been so kind to the whole family. Seeing him in concert at the O2 was an extraordinary evening to treasure.

Below right: The amazing Vickie White has shared the ups and downs and always helps to cheer me up.

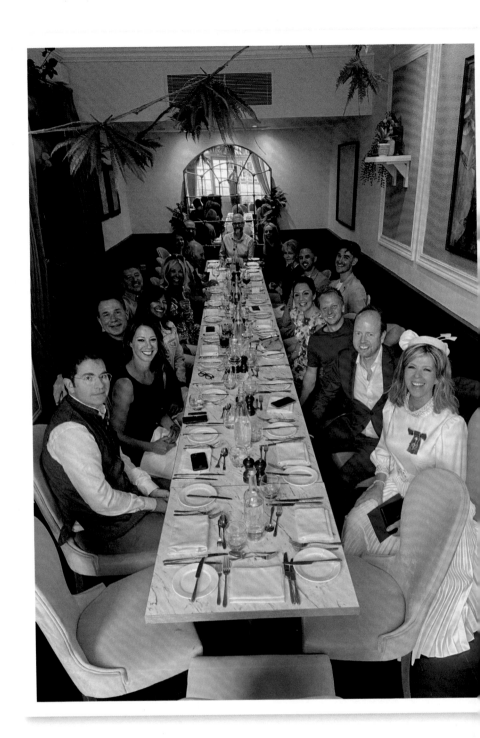

The love of friends, family and supportive bosses have been a lifeline to me. *Clockwise from bottom left*: Ben Wegg-Prosser, Gloria de Piero, Richard Arnold, Ranvir Singh, Ben Shephard, Vickie White, my dad, Gordon, Clare Holt, John Chittenden, James Daniel, Sally Ardis, my mum, Marylyn, James Delamare, Tom Kehoe, Laura Tobin, Matt Nicholls, Max Dundas – and me!

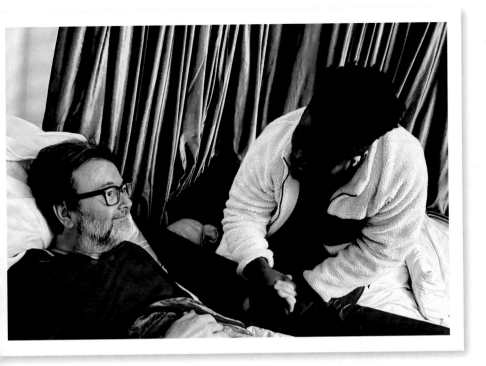

Derek's carers move me so much in their dedication and compassion –
Jake Sackey has been working with him for over a year.

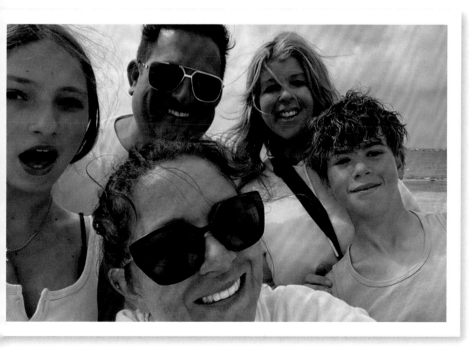

Chris Hawkins and Clare Nasir have been so supportive to me. Darcey took
this photo just after the swim that gave me perspective. Also pictured are Chris
and Clare's daughter (and my god-daughter) Sienna, and Billy.

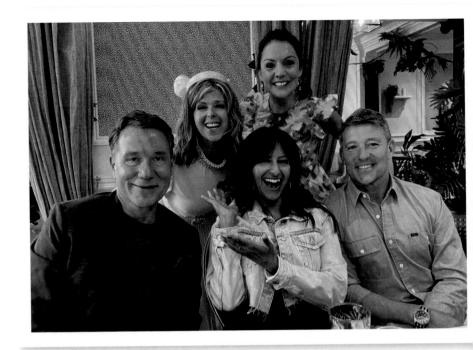

Ben Shephard, Richard Arnold, Ranvir Singh, Laura Tobin and I have a bond forged over many years of working (and playing!) together in the wee small hours. We've shared so many life-changing moments that we feel like family.

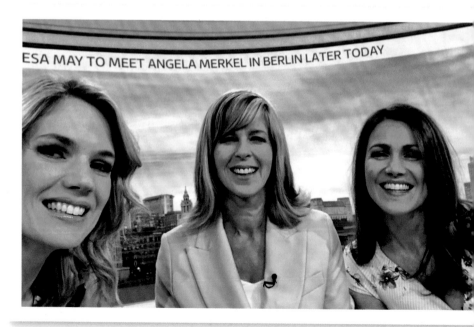

ESA MAY TO MEET ANGELA MERKEL IN BERLIN LATER TODAY

Having supportive work colleagues is vital. Charlotte has stepped in at short notice when I've had to rush to Derek's side and Susanna even gave up her own holiday once to cover for me.

Chapter 6

Sharking It

We knew Derek's body had been wracked with Covid and we knew his brain had been affected, too. Keeping him safe – alive – had always been the priority, but as the weeks turned into months and then into years, we realised that staying alive, simply existing, wasn't enough. Not for any of us – but most of all, not for Derek.

It sounds hideously ungrateful, and I feel guilty even saying it out loud, when so many lost their lives and others continue to fight for life in so many ways every day – and, of course, I know, life is everything. Where there is life, there is hope – that had been my mantra for so long. But life isn't just a bunch of chemical reactions in the body, is it? It isn't just organs and systems functioning adequately – lungs oxygenating, heart pumping, stomach processing, liver detoxifying, kidneys filtering and the rest of it – although these are all necessary to staying alive. Life and existence are different, though, aren't they? Living is like enjoying a fantastic meal with friends, whereas surviving is answering a belly growl of hunger with fuel.

Every morning, as the first rays of light filtered through the curtains in Derek's makeshift bedroom, I would sit quietly beside his bed, bracing myself for the same bittersweet ritual. Derek lay still, the silence broken only by his wrenching gasps for breath; even when he was in a deep sleep, his body seemed stiff, as if held captive by Covid.

As I watched him, my heart ached with a mixture of hope and despair, for I knew what would unfold when he awoke. His eyelids would flutter, like wings preparing for takeoff – the start of a new day, filled with all the promise and energy each morning used to bring for Derek. Slowly, ever so slowly, his eyes would open and, for a second, they would look like the eyes of the 'old Derek' – sleepy, but with all the old depth and knowledge. Then that expression would disappear like smoke in the wind, so I'd wonder if I had imagined it, and I'd witness cruel reality crashing down upon him: a torrential wave of profound disappointment. Etched in his new gaze would be a different kind of knowing – the realisation that he remained trapped within the confines of his own body.

As his eyes scanned the room, I imagined the echoes

of his dreams lingering in his mind. Perhaps in his slumber, he had inhabited the life we'd had before – the effortless laughter, the touch of his fingertips, the easy hugs with his children, the words he used to weave into eloquent tales, the sharpness of his mind. But as consciousness dawned, the stark contrast between his dreams and his waking reality was painfully revealed. The weight of his paralysis descended upon him, the heavy shroud of his near-silent existence.

It was in those solitary moments, in the intimate witnessing of his awakening each morning, that I confronted the depths of my own sadness. Yet this daily ritual both shattered and fortified my spirit, for amid the profound sadness was a renewed determination to be his voice, to bridge the gap between his thoughts and the world. And that always rallied me.

But I couldn't just speak for him and move mountains for him, however hard I might want to try. Yes, we could navigate the uncharted territory of his altered existence together but, ultimately, I could see in his eyes that I had to somehow help him be the captain of his own ship – as much as he could be. In the unspoken language of our shared journey, for him to begin to break free I knew I had to find a way to help him unlock his own prison because that's how he would truly start living, even within the restrictions of his disability. Derek needed to feel a sense of progress.

Living life on a rollercoaster, as we were – and still

are – we could celebrate the ups, however small they might be, and treasure the joy of an hour together that we thought we would never see. But to get through the downs, we had to have an eye on the horizon, a fixed point in the future, where the ride would somehow even out – where the dips would be shallower, the highs less steep – where we could coast for a bit or rest on a ledge before moving on. And we hoped those times would extend from a few minutes to a few hours, to a whole day, without plunging into a dip or moving backwards, and that the ups would begin to last longer.

My friend, Piers Morgan, always quotes Winston Churchill: 'If you're going through hell, keep going.' In other words, 'Don't stop and take up residence in hell, don't accept the horrible place you're in as the norm. Keep going, in the certainty that at some point there will be an end, an outcome, a place you will reach, because the very act of keeping going is healing, in a way that giving up never can be.'

Derek once had his own version of this; he used to talk about 'sharking it', because some shark species, including the Great White, need to keep swimming and filtering water through their gills just to stay alive. If these sharks stop swimming, they lose oxygen and die, so they have to keep moving forward. The action of movement has an innate purpose – you either keep going or die.

Derek has always been big on purpose as a drive for really living. He wrote about it in his book, *Create Space*, and in his psychology articles, where he argued that it was one of the vital components for good mental health – for people generally and for him personally. He realised that a lot of his work in politics was about the drive to do some good, which gave him a sense of purpose in his own life. After he left politics, he had gone on to find purpose in the mental health and coaching work he'd been doing since I had known him.

He used to say that when you have a purpose and a goal, painful, difficult or boring tasks seem less so. They can bring you joy despite the tedium, because you know you're doing them for a reason. You can hold in your mind why you are doing them and the 'why' justifies the hardship of the 'what' and the 'how'. When we first met, he'd already worked in businesses and set up several companies. He would say, 'In business you can't stay still, Kate. You expand or die.'

So it wasn't enough just to keep Derek alive. We had to keep 'sharking it', striving to get him better, never doubting it was possible, because in the act of striving and keeping going we were doing something, not just waiting for it to happen to us. We were making each day better, giving each day purpose.

Without a sense of purpose, without a sense of growth, none of us can tolerate the uncertainty of the day to day, can we? We turn in on ourselves, we overanalyse, we allow hopelessness and despair to take over. Action, though, always generates a reaction in those around

The Strength of Love

us: it creates ripples, it creates energy. And I believe positive action creates positive vibrations, if only because taking action stops us from worrying and fretting. This approach seems to work whatever the challenge we face, be it financial, emotional or health-related.

So we had to keep moving towards Derek getting better, for our sake and for his sake too – to bolster *our* spirit. To sustain us all through the ups and downs, we needed to believe that there was some kind of safe and contented place for us to reach for somewhere on the horizon.

Derek called the first company he set up after we met 'Flow'. The name was inspired by the book, *Flow: The Psychology of Optimal Experience* by Mihaly Csikszentmihalyi, a Hungarian-American psychologist. Published in 1990, the book explores the concept of flow, referring to a state of complete focus and immersion in an activity, and how that immersion can in itself lead to joy and happiness – or at least that was how Derek interpreted it and how he used it in his psychology work with teams and individuals.

To get to this state of flow, you need to have a clear objective or goal in mind and fully immerse yourself in the process of achieving it. Because you are intensely focused on the task at hand, you stop worrying and fretting about other things and this gives you a sense of control or mastery, which releases serotonin and literally creates joy in the brain.

If there is a good balance between the level of the challenge and the skill required to do the task, you can get a sense of satisfaction. If the task is too easy, it can lead to boredom; if too difficult, it can result in anxiety or frustration. So if it's too hard for you, you will feel like a failure; but if it's too easy, it won't test you enough to give you a sense of achievement when it's completed. This is what we had to do with Derek – find a way of caring for him that gave a sense of progress as well as simply keeping him alive.

As we cared for him, I tried to break down the different barriers that were holding him back, to see if we could fill his day with 'tasks', activities that would give him 'purpose' on top of the continuous caring tasks he needed us to carry out to keep him alive. Yes, there was muscle weakness; yes, there was organ damage; yes, there were breathing challenges and infection risk; but there was something else too. The hospital had said he had difficulty 'initiating' and this related to movement and speech. Basically, he couldn't connect his thoughts – what he wanted to do or say – to his body, whether due to nerve damage or weakness. They hoped the ability was in there, we just had to find a key to unlock it.

For this process of initiating, rehabilitation is crucial because it triggers something called 'brain plasticity', meaning the brain's ability to rewire itself. By repeating things again and again – movements and words – the brain can reconnect and start 'talking to' arms and legs

159

and vocal cords, and enable the person to walk and speak again. We had no idea whether this would be possible with Derek because there were so many unknowns, but at least it gave us something tangible to aim for.

On Derek's release, the hospital specialists insisted to the community teams that he would need ongoing rehabilitation, so that he didn't regress. I say rehabilitation, but it was officially called 'therapeutic input to optimise disability'. Catchy, huh?!! This was because they had no way of knowing if Derek could improve and regain any movement or speech, so they didn't want to set unrealistic expectations. But neither, mercifully, did they see it as palliative. We took some hope from that – he hadn't been written off – but everyone said not to expect too much and kept on telling Derek the same too. I banned this. 'Why shouldn't he rehabilitate and get back more of himself?' I said.

I may have over-egged it in order to offset more than a year of negativity and fear, of hanging onto life by a thread, but I wanted him to feel empowered. I felt it was this fire that had helped him to survive Covid's onslaught so far – and now more than ever he needed to reignite that fighting spirit.

I chose not to say 'optimise disability' to Derek, but 'rehabilitate', because the word meant progress to me. Rehabilitation, in its broadest sense, is defined as the process of restoring someone or something to a healthy, functional or improved state. Yes, it actually means improved! There seemed to me so much promise in this definition!

My friend, Penny Stokes Hilton, who is an estate agent (or realtor, as they are called in the US), inspired me even more when she explained how Americans view rehab in relation to buildings. They use it in the sense of restoration, renovation and improvement. Not just getting a building back to the way it was but making it even better! They see a rehab as an upgrade to enhance a property and its value.

I loved this! When I told Derek that this was a chance to be even better than he was before, he would whisper, 'I will do it, I can do it', and it felt as if we were turning around the negatives of the past year – the warnings of death, of no chance of recovery – and focusing on striving to get better and have a brighter future. A different future, of course, but no less good.

So I chose to think of Derek's therapeutic input as rehabilitation. I've now learned that terms like 'intervention to optimise disability' are used to help the care system allocate resources. In other words, if someone has a chance of getting better, it's worth investing in rehab, but then they don't get ongoing care support. If the person gets rehab, they are not supposed to need long-term care and support, because they're going to get better. But it's a terrible Catch-22 if you're in a situation like Derek's.

We knew that it would take time for him to get better

– and that he might not get better at all – but we had to push that out of our minds and embrace the chance of rehabilitation in its most positive sense. This meant focusing less on our anxiety about what could go wrong with our care of Derek and more on what could go right.

We didn't know if he could improve, but the specialists had stressed to the community teams that his care wasn't about 'giving up' and 'just making Derek comfortable'. So we grabbed any help we could. We felt as if we'd snatched Derek from the jaws of death, so the idea of keeping him here with us and 'optimising' what we could felt like a gift from the gods. I told myself and Derek, 'You have already defied the odds. You can defy this too and improve.'

Rehab gave us hope that this wasn't *it*, that this hanging between life and death wasn't forever. We had purpose and forward motion.

The rehab he could get in hospital was limited by his condition and fatigue. In the community, perhaps unsurprisingly, it was much more limited by resources and available staff; there was so much pressure on the system and we were grateful for whatever help they could give us.

Derek had been released from hospital because they could not keep him there, due to a Covid outbreak. We'd hoped that the rehab they'd been doing in the hospital – which seemed so promising – could continue at home. But I quickly realised that, when it comes to therapy in the community, trained therapists are very limited so the programme essentially relies on training others – such as carers and relatives – to help with exercises that the person can then learn to do on their own.

Clearly, this would be almost impossible to achieve with Derek, because of his extreme vulnerability and the variability of his condition. It was a huge ask for the carers to take on the responsibility of trying to help him improve, especially when there were still so many gaps in the specialists' knowledge about exactly what might be holding him back – and I couldn't do it alone because there always needed to be at least two people present. It took weeks of assessment, but we were finally allocated a rehab team – an occupational therapist and a physiotherapist – who could come at least once a fortnight.

I felt sorry for some of the therapists when they first arrived because you could see in their eyes that they were overwhelmed by the task they'd been given. It was like trying to fit a square peg in a round hole, because they had to try to fit Derek's needs to what they could offer, rather than being able to offer him what he needed. You could see it pained them to be forced to approach it this way.

For the OT, it was particularly challenging. If you've never had any need for an OT, you might not know what they do. Essentially, they are brilliant, skilled people who help you learn how to make your life work again. In the hospital, this literally means working out what you can and can't do – for example, seeing if you can learn to wash yourself or make your own cup of tea. In the process, they help you understand the boundaries of your new condition. OTs in the community help you set up your home appropriately and, if you're lucky enough to still be able to work, they show you how to manage in the short term and work out what is best in the long term. Essentially, they help you get your life back on track.

In the community, the OT usually works with the carers to help the person maximise what they can do; the aim, of course, is that they will eventually need less care. And this was what we wanted too; this approach is also clearly much better financially for society. As we all know, care is in short supply and super-costly.

However, Derek wasn't able to do what the OTs needed him to be able to do in the time period we had been allocated. The carers became increasingly frustrated. They kept saying, 'The therapists want us to do this and do that, but we can't. It's unsafe; Derek isn't strong or stable enough and we're not physically strong enough to be able to do it with him, either.'

I could see that the carers were right. It needed a very experienced therapist to know exactly where to put their hand on Derek's back, or where to put their foot behind his heel to make sure he could put some pressure in the right areas to begin to understand the sensation of being more upright and so start getting his limbs and brain to talk to each other again. Without the help of someone with the right level of knowledge and experience, he would end up flopping down in a precarious position, potentially harming himself, the carers, the kids and me.

The safest place to keep him was flat on his back in bed. But this wasn't a helpful solution either because it increased the risk of pressure sores forming on his limbs. This then increased the risk of his skin becoming infected, which in turn increased the risk of all kinds of complications and setbacks, including not being able to move at all, leading to even worse pressure sores. Yet another vicious circle. I began to see that nothing was without risk: staying still wasn't an option and we had to push the envelope to go forward or we would go back. We had to expand or die! Not least because our care support package was always in jeopardy.

Most long-term care, in my experience, is very hard to secure. And when it is refused, it is left to the individual to battle, with appeals funded at their own cost, to prove what is seemingly obvious to those at the coalface – that the care is in fact vital. So, when you do have a care package in place, knowing that it's temporary can make you feel like you've got a ticking time bomb under your chair; there's this ever present panic in your chest that the care could be taken away at any minute, exploding your world and obliterating any sense of safety. Worrying about it makes you feel that everything is a race against time – and then you're back to relying on our friend adrenaline to get you through, from minute to minute, hour to hour.

We hit a low one day when even our incredibly supportive local authority ran out of time. They had been desperately trying to give us some support while we waited for the appeal board to get back to us with a date for our hearing, but now they said they simply could not continue to support us. The person on the end of the phone was deeply emotional about having to deliver this terrible news, and told me that they were trying to organise at least some carers' 'visits' to check on Derek when I had to leave the house. I said this would be unsafe: Derek couldn't be left alone because of the risk to himself. The only thing they could offer us was a crash mat in case he fell out of bed.

I said this wouldn't work because he was liable to do himself serious damage. This was aside from the emotional impact a catastrophe like falling out of bed would have on someone like Derek, who was already psychologically very vulnerable and, the carers said, becoming increasingly desperate at his plight when I wasn't around.

One of the biggest problems was that Derek's day-to-day condition was so dramatically unpredictable. He wasn't in the same bracket as, say, a friend of ours who had come home after a minor stroke and was on an established path to recovery. Not that I'm downplaying the challenges he faced, of course; it's just that this was a whole different kind of challenge for which professional care was vital.

We continued to wait for the appeal date to be set and, while we did, I decided that we might as well grab the best advice from the OT team while we could.

The OTs wanted to talk about where we could position rails that, in the future, might help Derek to manoeuvre himself in the specially adapted shower we had installed. I knew this was at least months and possibly years away, if ever, but also knew that I wanted to be positive and look to the future.

We bought the rails and booked in a team from the local authority to install them, as that gave us more confidence that it would be done correctly; they came and drilled holes in the wall, ready to put the rails in, and said they would be back. But then our local authority support ran out and it was decided that, as Derek was nowhere near needing the rails, they wouldn't be able to come back to fit them. I refused to give up, though. I just thought, 'We'll need them one day. I'm leaving the holes there … One day he will be that strong and we can get someone back to fit those rails.'

It took several weeks for the physio team to come and assess Derek, by which point we had observed that he would always try his best to move himself when we were moving him, even though he was so weak and at times in so much pain that he had tears rolling down his face.

The therapist who had worked with him in the hospital had also noticed this. She said that he had never once refused to do therapy when asked, and seemed brighter when trying to activate and strengthen his muscles. So I had high hopes that he would respond well when the physiotherapy started again.

When we told him that the time had come when we could have physiotherapy at home, he looked uplifted, even delighted. They were a brilliant team: so overstretched and under-resourced, but fighting to do their best, and it felt as if Derek's spirit was rising with every session. If I told him in the morning that the physios were coming later that day, he'd smile and whisper, 'When, when?' His ability to judge time was very poor, so he would go on asking every few minutes, 'When? When?' until they arrived.

He was too weak to move at all at first and we initially had to gently see if he could move any of his limbs, even slightly. This involved lots of stretching and we were carefully shown how to help him with this; I could see he was in agony at times and disorientated at others; but he kept going, kept trying. It was clear how much it meant to him to be pushing himself towards recovery – he was doing it for us and also for himself.

The physio came with an assistant (while the carer was also there), and I carefully watched what the physio did so I could understand how he was moving Derek safely. When the physios were there, it was incredible.

They gave us all a sense that we were cracking on. Derek responded every single time, no matter how painful a struggle it was, pushing himself to the limit until he was shaking all over. The children would whoop and cheer as they watched him make each slight movement, spurring him on and boosting his determination; you could sense him coming out of himself. He would often have to sleep for three hours afterwards to recover energy and strength.

I already knew something about physical rehab after meeting a former soldier whose arms had been blown off by an explosive device. He'd had two incredible arm transplants – he was the first person in the world to be given two limb transplants at the same time, and was undergoing rehab in France when I met him. I've interviewed him several times during his journey and he's always inspiring. At our most recent meeting, he'd said that he had started to get more use of his arms and hands. For the transplants to 'take', he explained, he had to 'get the nerves to talk to his hands' and, after nine months, that conversation was beginning to happen. The doctors had warned him that, if it worked at all, it would be at least two years, but he was having none of it! He wanted it to happen more quickly.

'How did you do it?' I asked, 'And ahead of schedule, as well?'

'Repetitive, boring, unbelievably exhausting rehab, nine hours a day,' he replied.

Sometimes, he said, he would do the same thing with his fingers, just up and down, again and again, and again, *and again*, never stopping to rest. But that was better than the alternative, he said, which was the nothingness of waiting. He also felt he had been given such a chance with the transplants that he wanted to make good the work of others.

I knew Derek suffered from guilt. He'd get emotional at times, thinking of those who had lost their lives to Covid. When I tried to lift his spirits by saying what a miracle it was that he'd come through, he would say, 'But what about the people who died?'

I would cheerlead and say, 'You have to make it count, don't you? And keep going for those who haven't had the chance.' In his moments of greater consciousness, he would understand this and slowly nod.

The first time the physio had come, he positioned Derek upright with his legs dangling over the end of the bed; he needed two people behind to keep him upright and the physio supporting from the front. Derek's eyes were wide open and I could see his fear; I can only imagine what was going through his mind after a year and a half of being flat. Coming into an upright position, even just sitting, must have been terrifying. Did he feel a sense of vertigo? Dizziness? We had to be alert to any sign of a drop in his blood pressure, which they'd observed had happened during physio in the hospital. We didn't have a way of monitoring that at home, but it was a factor in our thinking. If his blood pressure dropped dramatically, he could pass out, and where would that lead? What damage could it do? We had no way of telling.

The physio encouraged us to use the manual hoist, as it meant he could be up in a sort of sitting position in a safe way. We have large mirrors in our sitting room – now his bedroom – and as we wheeled him round to face them, I was anxiously looking at him, checking his feet were in position and everything else was in place. He was up high, almost as if he were standing upright at his full six foot two, and, as I looked up at his face, I realised he was staring straight ahead at the mirror. I turned to look in the mirror, too – and there we were, a couple – with me, at five foot two, next to him.

At that moment I realised – and it hit me like a punch in the face – that I hadn't been in this position, almost standing next to him, since the day he went into hospital. I'd gone from his bedside looking down at him, lying flat, to occasionally sitting next to him, propped up in bed, to washing him in the adapted shower room – but now we were 'standing' together. It could've been our wedding day. It could've been the day we carried Darcey or Billy out of hospital.

The silence was thick. He just stared, wide-eyed, at his own reflection and then looked at my reflection, too.

Without thinking I gently linked my arm through his, like in our wedding snaps.

He started to cry. 'I want this!' he exclaimed.

He didn't have to say what he wanted – I knew. He wanted life, not existence, and he wanted his old self back again and the old us back and to stand tall, with me by his side.

'You are my husband and we are "us", whether you are sitting or standing, darling,' I said. 'But I know why you want it for *you*.'

I knew he couldn't find the words to express the overwhelming surge of emotions flooding his heart. But he knew he didn't have to. Together, we simply lived the moment in silence. He hung on to the bar on the hoist, keeping himself upright for as long as he could – nearly ten minutes, his longest ever – his muscles trembling with effort.

But there was a fire in his vulnerability. The image I saw in the mirror was a reflection of his extraordinary resilience, his fight, and the unyielding part of his spirit.

And my heart soared, too.

* * *

I held that image in my mind as we ploughed on, 'sharking it', always one step forward two steps back, but constantly edging on.

One of the biggest barriers to seeing any real progress was overwhelming fatigue that would just stop Derek dead in his tracks. One specialist confided that while they had learned so much more about how to mitigate the worst of the symptoms of Covid since Derek contracted it in 2020 – and of course the vaccines had been developed to prevent and reduce suffering – the chronic fatigue was still largely a mystery.

Was it his blood pressure dropping, or a failure in the autonomic system? Was it a problem with his digestive system, or the recurrent infections at the PEG site and other areas? Or something more sinister, damage as yet undetected? We couldn't know.

I tried to research what the fatigue might be. I thought it was probably a combination of everything and I desperately pushed for referrals to different specialists, thinking that if we could improve every bit of him that was damaged – the liver, the kidney, the heart, the lungs and all – then maybe that small degree of improvement in each area would have a cumulative effect. Years later, when Derek's referrals for the long Covid clinic finally came up, I was reassured that my instincts had been right. That's exactly how the experts there began approaching the problem.

One piece of research I did in my quest to find out as much as I could about every part of Derek's condition was about how the mitochondria in every cell are often left damaged after Covid. The damage was described as like the batteries of the post-Covid cell never quite fully recharging and on top of that, losing power far too quickly. 'That's exactly Derek!' I thought. Research in this area is still so limited and there are few experts in this field, but we are hoping to get to see someone soon.

Friends offered help, too – love stretching out its long fingers. Penny Smith, my friend from *GMTV*, got in touch and said she'd been reading about treatments abroad that she thought might work; she also wanted to put me in contact with another presenter with whom we'd both worked in the past. This presenter's daughter had suffered a severe brain injury and, after long months of rehabilitation, needed more support after being discharged. She had found that neuro-training worked really well and I followed up to see if it might be helpful for Derek. Even though at the time he was too weak to benefit fully from it, we're using it again now and I genuinely think it is helping his focus.

Another friend, life coach Pete Cohen, whose wife was seriously ill at the time, got in touch to tell me about the importance of diet. It blew me away that he cared so much to try to help Derek, even when he had his own huge troubles to deal with. He put me in touch with a nutritionist in Sweden who used specific supplements to aid people who'd had long spells in intensive care and suffered from severe inflammation of the organs and nervous system. He set about drafting a list of supplements that he believed would benefit Derek. We had to have a whole range of new and unusual blood tests done before we could consider giving any to Derek and these threw up an unusual result ... Derek's blood was incredibly acidic, an indicator that he may not be breathing out enough carbon dioxide. Investigations into his breathing so far had looked at the damage to the lining of his lungs and the transfer of oxygen across it. But exhaling carbon dioxide is less to do with that, and more to do with the diaphragm. Derek's diaphragm was weakened, and holding onto carbon dioxide can be almost as damaging as not getting enough oxygen.

So a blood test to look for nutritional deficiency had now led to Derek being put on the waiting list for respiratory rehab that may well lead to the break-through in fatigue which we were hoping for in the first place!

For Derek, though, none of these breakthroughs could come fast enough. While we waited for the poor overstretched doctors and nurses to clear the backlog, it seemed Derek's attempts to get upright and walk had hit a dead end. That moment in the mirror now almost seemed like a wonderful mirage.

Some friends worried that all this advice was leading me down blind alleys, raising false hope and exhausting me in the meantime, but I found that even when the suggestions didn't necessarily lead to immediate answers, they threw up new ideas and perspectives, which then continued to take us forward, with the momentum of purpose.

Despite the physio's hope that simple stretching would help release the contractions of Derek's muscles and ligaments from months of lying prone, this was not to be. He couldn't get upright to use his body weight to stretch through his legs because he couldn't balance. And he couldn't balance because his legs and feet were contracted. It was a vicious circle.

The experts suggested looking at some contraptions to help gently stretch the muscles and ligaments. One such device was fitted over and behind his knee and down to his shins and over the back of his heel. It looked like some kind of Victorian caliper and, each day, we had to tighten screws to increase the tension. He needed to wear these for at least 12 hours a day so the obvious time to put them on was in the evening and at night. He didn't really like wearing them as they made lying flat so awkward and uncomfortable, and I worried because it looked so miserable and so painful, like having a constant cramp you couldn't ease.

Sometimes, at night, he would wake up and I would relieve the tension for a while by releasing the screws so that he could sleep better. The next day, though, he would say to me, 'Why did you do that? I want them to work.' And I couldn't help but admire his perseverance.

After weeks and months of this, there were very small improvements and an orthopaedic expert was drafted in. He took one look at Derek's legs with his knees in a permanent bent position and pointing like a ballerina's and said that no amount of contractions or stretching exercises were going to solve this, and that he needed surgery to ease the tension. To illustrate this, he got me to stand up on my tiptoes, with my knees bent and asked me to hold the position. I couldn't! He pointed out that if I couldn't do it when I was fit and healthy and strong, then what must it be like for Derek, considering all the other problems he had?

He was put on the waiting list and when the time came for the operation, he faced it bravely. It meant weeks in plaster and in pain for it to heal, and then he had to begin the whole process of strengthening his muscles again.

After the surgery on his legs, he was recommended for inpatient rehab, which went incredibly well, but he wasn't able to complete it because a new infection sent him back into intensive care to fight for his life all over again.

Frustratingly, Derek had been complaining of back pain during the rehab but it was assumed that was down to him being moved more. Unfortunately, the cause was far more serious and it was to do with his kidneys. Somehow, because of all the different hospitals Derek had been transferred to and all the different specialist departments he was under, it had been missed that, since contracting Covid, he had been developing kidney stones. I now know that the dialysis that Derek had needed is a vital, life-saving piece of kit but is nowhere near as good at keeping everything working as healthy kidneys. I've been told that it's very common to develop kidney stones following dialysis. Amid the drama of the many things Derek's doctors were up against, the appropriate scan hadn't taken place and the kidney stones had been left to develop over the last few years. His tubes were now so blocked that his system was being poisoned.

He had come home for a visit and within hours he started to shake, his temperature going through the roof. We called our GP, who said he would come out as soon as he finished surgery. But then, as the shaking worsened, he told us to call an ambulance immediately.

It was terrifying, and a fearful echo of the day he was taken away with Covid. The carer and I feared the worst, but at least this time there were no restrictions so I could go in the ambulance with him.

He was gasping in pain as the ambulance raced to the hospital. I tried to keep calm as I wondered what could be threatening to take him away from us this time.

'This time I'm a goner, Kate,' he said.

I squeezed his hand hard. 'You are not. You've come this far, you are not leaving us now. Fight for it.'

When we arrived, the doctors tried a process of elimination to work out what was wrong. His blood pressure was plummeting dramatically and they quickly identified that he had severe sepsis. The challenge was to find the cause – until you know that there is no way to begin treating it. The doctors warned us that it was a race against time and that it was 50-50 as to whether he'd make it through the night. By now, it was 1am, and a whole group of doctors were trying to figure out which organ was failing and where the infection stemmed from. Then one junior doctor asked me, 'What did you think it might be when you called the ambulance?' I said I didn't really know, but that I thought it might be a urine infection as he was prone to those. Strangely, though, he hadn't been passing any urine. The doctors looked at each other and said in unison, 'Kidneys.' The kidney stones had blocked his tubes and he was operated on straight away. Drains were put in his kidneys and, over the next week, we waited nervously as the pus and infection were drained out.

Yet again, he had defied the odds and the medical team had performed a miracle. It meant that he had to remain in intensive care for weeks, of course, and was then moved to another hospital to begin the process of recovering and gaining strength once more.

Again, we had to fight to safely bring him home and Derek had to find the strength to restart the healing process. This time, though, there was a difference. Derek had shown us that he had the capacity to surprise and thrive, despite all the odds. It was a miraculous moment. Looking back, it seems so extraordinary. If it wasn't recorded in the therapist's notes, I might not have believed what I'd seen.

Before sepsis had taken him back to intensive care, we had taken Derek into the hall to try to get him to bear weight by holding the stair banisters, because his arms had become stronger and he was able to move them and squeeze his hands to grip better.

'Upstairs,' he suddenly said.

'What do you mean, upstairs?' I asked.

'Want to go,' he said, as though it was taking all his strength just to draw in the breath to get the words out.

Upstairs? It seemed impossible. But Derek's parents and his sister happened to be in the house, as well as the kids and the physio and his assistant. I looked at the physio, who was with us for the final visit of our allotted sessions and was sad because he didn't want this to be his last day. I knew what he was thinking. It was the first time Derek had expressed a desire to break free and, as the timer had run out on physio visits, it was now or never.

'How do we do this?' he said under his breath. He looked over at me and said, 'Okay, I know.'

He and the assistant put their full body weight behind Derek's legs and the carers stood above. We watched in disbelief as Derek painfully hauled himself up the stairs with pushes and pulls, accompanied by screams of delight from the kids and his parents.

After six stairs, there is a mini landing in our house. We carried the wheelchair up and he rested. I gave him a feed of high sugar nutrition and some water through his PEG, as I could see he was flaked, maybe even broken. We looked at each other and wondered how on earth we were going to get him down, but all I said was, 'You are amazing, Derek.

He looked at me and, in barely a whisper said, 'Keep going.'

I think privately we all wondered if it was wise, but he seemed so definite, so determined, that no one wanted to break the euphoria of this extraordinary moment. We were all following *his* lead.

Suddenly he was empowered. He was taking control and he didn't want to let go. There were only three more steps, and somehow we got him up them. His sisters were above and quickly grabbed the chair. We helped him sit down and he looked around.

I suddenly realised that he hadn't been upstairs since the day he had left our house in March 2020 in an ambulance, and at the same time realised what a state the upstairs was in! Derek was always so organised. His study, right next to the top of the stairs, was so neat, everything in its place.

'Oh my God, you're going to say that I've let your study get into a mess,' I said.

He craned his head to the right to try to see. The jokey sign on the outside door of his study said 'Operations Room' and I recalled how many times I had looked at this sign while he was in hospital, wondering if he would ever speak again, recognise us, feel our love and be able to express his. Wondering if he'd even survive at all.

The four of us carefully shifted the wheelchair round and I opened the door. Darcey was squealing in delight. 'Dad, Dad, what do you think of what Mum's done to your study?'

He looked in and smiled, a long, slow smile, and then,

almost as if he was cranking his neck back, he looked Darcey and Billy hard in the face and said, 'Shameful.'

We all burst into tears, including Derek. It was such a Derek word – he would always look at things and joke and say 'shameful' or 'disgraceful' to me, especially when he was teasing me for being untidy. And he said it in such a way, with a hint of a Lancashire accent that instantly connected us all to his familiar humour. 'Shaaaaaymful.'

I felt as though I had taken some kind of hallucinogenic drug. Even the physio and his assistant's eyes welled up.

'He's back!' said Billy. 'My dad is back!'

To this day, Derek still has not managed to go upstairs again. But he'd done it once; his spirit and his fight had got him up those stairs. It had been his purpose and he had to see it through. Now that he'd done it once, we knew that he knew he could do it again. I was determined to keep searching for more, to keep trying everything I possibly could that might help him in his fight. We had to keep going – we just had to keep sharking it.

Chapter 7

A Leap of Faith

All the glimpses of the 'old' Derek and the treasured memories of our past together made it impossible for me to do nothing while we waited for the specialist referrals he needed. These referrals were still at least a year away, and the coming 12 months would, I knew, be crucial to Derek's recovery and state of mind; we had to keep going forward, no matter what. I started looking around for other possibilities and treatments – anything at all that could help him improve – while trying to stay cautious about the more outlandish suggestions that sometimes came up.

Once the two documentaries we made, *Finding Derek* and *Caring for Derek*, had aired, it was wonderful to see how moved people were and they reached out to help. It was a flicker of light in the darkness, as people recognised his name and our story through my work on television and radio, and the ripple effect was incredible. It took my breath away, too, how many people in the health world urged us to keep going – not only practitioners of conventional medicine but also a whole range of alternative and natural health therapists and healers. It seemed Derek's spirit had touched the hearts of strangers and their response to it was like a gust of wind propelling us forward when we needed it most. We had slowed down and become becalmed, in a way, since Derek had climbed the stairs that day – despite the daily frenzied activity needed to keep him alive. And now we had a new power in our sails to spur us on again.

'Keep the ship afloat,' I would say to myself in moments of exhaustion, when I just didn't know how I was going to keep going and keep our spirits up.

It was isolating at times, too. The practical realities of caring mean you have little time for 'normal' socialising and friendship – and anyway I didn't want to bother the wonderful people around me, who I knew had troubles of their own. At these times, our ship felt stranded, sequestered by fear and illness, but then bottles would wash up from the outside world with messages of hope.

People got in touch to pass on information about what had helped them and I resolved to look at it all when I had a second: how hyperbaric oxygen chambers had been shown by Israeli researchers to be having a positive effect on Covid patients; how Reiki, which was something Derek believed in, could be restorative. A producer I worked with on *Strictly Come Dancing* years ago got in touch, saying her life had been changed by Pranic healing, which we then began to explore; and we also learned about remote healing, which is practised at a distance and sounds far-fetched, but a lot of people swear by it. I heard about experimental treatments and clinical trials in new therapies from around the world. It was wonderful to see how, even though the national and global Covid emergency was no longer daily headline news, the medical profession kept pressing on to search for a cure, for the disease itself and also for the damage it causes. I was reminded that, of course, they did this every day, with every disease and ailment – and it's humbling.

Some of the information I was given came from people who were directly affected by Covid; others wanted to share lessons they had learned while fighting for loved ones who had other long-term conditions in case that might help Derek and our family. I believe all these contacts were powered by the force of love, coming from a place where they wanted to find a purpose in their suffering: by sharing with me what they had discovered, they were sharing their love, their struggles and their pain. They were connecting. I resolved that if I learned anything useful in my research, I would share it with them in turn, and with the medical profession.

Of course, I didn't want to do anything that would further risk Derek's health, however promising the recommendations might sound. But I also increasingly wondered if doing nothing posed risks too. Progress stagnating seemed to be increasingly dispiriting for Derek and it wasn't as though simply keeping him alive day-to-day was easy. I felt if I relaxed for a moment, something would be missed or a new infection would set in. Nothing felt truly *safe*.

Simply waiting for referrals and tests felt increasingly like a dangerous game, as crucial details continued to fall through the cracks. For this I don't in any way blame the medical professionals who faced the challenge of Derek's unprecedented and intricate case. I felt *for* them, because it must have been like trying to grasp a blancmange that was constantly slipping through their fingers. Each time they thought they had a handle on one aspect of his condition, it became painfully clear that other, hidden factors were at play. Clarity eluded us as we desperately sought a definitive diagnosis and tried to unravel the true impact of Covid on Derek's ravaged body and brain. All we could do was piece together the scattered clues and respond accordingly.

Determined to find something, anything, that could offer a glimmer of hope in the meantime, I felt we needed to make a leap of faith and try something new.

One suggestion that came in was for treatment in Mexico. Everything about it seemed fated: this new treatment was an American project, but one of the directors on the team was Welsh and often came back to the UK to see his family; he happened to be here the week our documentary, *Finding Derek*, was broadcast; he saw it and showed it to the lead neurologist on the project and they thought they could help Derek.

He tried to get in touch, but by then Derek was back in hospital and I was struggling to keep on top of even the basics, let alone follow up anything new. The director didn't give up, though, because he gathered from the documentary that time was of the essence for the treatment to be most effective, so he spoke to a friend who spoke to another friend and eventually the message made its way to Charlotte Hawkins at *GMB*. I will never forget the day she told me about it and gave me his number; I don't know whether it was because it was her – I totally believe anything she tells me as she's so wonderfully organised and kind – or because the treatment seemed to offer exactly what Derek needed at that moment. It felt as if it was what I had been praying for.

So, yes, I decided to take a leap of faith, but of course I still had to do my due diligence first. You know me, always the journalist! I spoke directly to the lead doctor, who showed me videos of other people he'd helped with this treatment. They had different conditions, of course, because Covid was so new, but he explained to me why he believed Derek's situation might be similar to people he had successfully treated before. I also spoke to some of his patients directly and found that their cases had extraordinary echoes of Derek's.

These people had exhausted all available conventional medical options so were prepared to take part in clinical trials. I could tell they'd been desperate – they just knew they couldn't go on with a 'wait and see' approach forever. They'd weighed up the risks and in some cases had been rewarded with extraordinary progress in their loved one's condition. Of course, doctors can't recommend anything until they have absolute certainty that it works but for these people and increasingly for Derek, time isn't their friend. The treatment being offered to Derek used principles that had been around for decades but hadn't been applied in this way so I was confident that it would do no harm – I just couldn't guarantee it would lead to the astonishing results that others had seen. Medicine has always been about trial and error (penicillin was discovered by accident), and of course waiting to see is the best approach generally. But there are so many individuals, people I talk to, or hear about from strangers in the street, or read about on my social media who feel they don't have time to wait, either because they can sense their loved ones slipping away – physically, or in spirit – or because they, as carers, feel they're at breaking point.

Time is often the enemy for carers. It is for me. I never have enough hours in the day to be present for Derek and the children; there is always some drama that prevents me from doing the things that would be better for me and my family in the long term because I have to take care of the urgent; and there's never time to properly take care of myself, which is so important.

Deep down, I knew I couldn't go on like this forever, working and caring around the clock and surviving on pure adrenaline. I've talked to so many carers, too who, like the sufferers themselves, eventually get ground down and despondent from the lack of progress. The weight eventually breaks them and I didn't want that to happen to me. Talking to those who had taken part in the experimental treatments in Mexico, I heard something different – an optimism – and that's when I realised something profound. Taking action, as long as it isn't harmful, and even when it seems like a shot in the dark, is a form of healing in itself. Doing nothing, that's the real enemy. It gnaws at your spirit, erodes your will to keep going, to survive, to thrive. So, with each step we took on this painful journey, we weren't just chasing a cure for Derek or a reversal of the damage to his body. We were fuelling the fire within us.

I knew, too, that Derek would support being involved in experimental research. He'd approved being in a trial when he very first had Covid, but he hadn't been accepted in time. Later, when he was in the coma, the research on his condition, doctors told me, had helped others and I knew this was a boost to him. Now, at last, he could be part of something that might help him directly. There were practical challenges, though. At this point, he hadn't even been out of the house, other than to go to the hospital in medical transport for tests or when he had setbacks. So the idea of flying him across the Atlantic was extreme!

I had Derek assessed for his capacity to fly safely and started talking to British Airways for our first visit and to American Airlines for a later trip. The airline industry had been decimated by Covid and many airline workers were in need of support, so it was extraordinary the way they bent over backwards to support Derek as much as they could. They couldn't have been more generous with their encouragement and practical help. Individual staff members made it clear that they had been moved by Derek's story: 'You helped my friend's mum when you said never give up hope', 'Your documentary gave comfort to my sister, who's a carer', 'Keep fighting the good fight'. It made me feel that I was doing some good and I felt less guilty about constantly having to ask for favours from everyone around me, when they had already done so much.

Because it was at trial stage, the treatment was free but, of course, there were still costs in providing the medical support we needed to make the journey and to ensure 24-hour care for Derek outside of the treatment while we were out there. And remember, in Mexico and the US you have to pay for everything in the healthcare system; they probably wouldn't even give you a junior aspirin without charging you for it – which is another reason to cherish and support our NHS.

I hired a nurse for the trip and wondered at the things you find out when you do this. Did you know, for instance, that there are nursing agencies specialising entirely in travel? I let the carers and support staff know that this was my intention and it blew me away when every single one of them said, 'Go for it, go for it', even though taking Derek away meant a total disruption to their working lives and possibly their incomes. And yet they said, 'Please do it. We can't stand to see Derek wasting away.'

I hoped that the care authorities would see it that way too because in my mind, taking him away meant removing the burden of caring for him in the UK, so surely that would be seen as a positive. Unfortunately, they took a different approach. When we returned home, exhausted but exhilarated, we found that somewhere in the chain of care administration – and I'm not blaming any one individual here, I think it's just the spider's web of miscommunication – they had cancelled Derek's care and challenged whether it could ever be reinstated.

So I suddenly, without warning, found myself completely alone in looking after Derek. I had to call my bosses and tell them I couldn't make it in to work. I was awake 24 hours a day until my begs and pleas were heard and some support was reinstated. It was a reminder of how vital care was for us to have any chance of keeping

Derek safe. I was so sleep-deprived because of the night-time disruptions, I had to ask Darcey to stay up so that I could have a rest (something I hated having to do) but I just needed someone to watch him until I could take over again. She didn't mind and did it willingly, but she was suffering too, and so were her studies. I didn't want to burden her like this, as the thing that kept her going was hoping to do well at school, and in her GCSE exams, poor girl. But what choice did we have? It was a painful few weeks but I know that there are hundreds of thousands more who know this agony too, and I resolved once again to campaign for more support for the care system.

Despite all this, there is absolutely no doubt in my mind that the trip to Mexico was 100 per cent worth it. In terms of the improvements it's given Derek, the jury is still out on how much medical progress he has made since the treatment, although the current MRI scans look very promising and people keep telling me how much better he is looking. But I can't say any more at this point because it's not my story to tell. The treatment is still in trial stage and when the doctor is ready to release the results, others will have the chance to make their own decisions. I also don't want to give people false hope by saying it's worked brilliantly for Derek, because I am still unclear as to whether any progress can be put down solely to this particular treatment. The lead doctor's hope and hypothesis is that it could be helpful for dementia and could aid recovery from many brain and neurological disorders, which of course would have huge implications for billions of people around the world. So again I don't want to raise false hope until the doctors have the stats to back it up.

I also can't give too many details about what exactly happened and what the treatment actually is, because there are non-disclosure agreements in place. But what I can tell you is that, when we got out there, I put myself through three days of the treatment first to make sure that it wasn't painful, or detrimental in any way to me. I also asked people in the medical profession, including doctors working with Derek in the UK, to analyse the treatment so that I knew it would cause absolutely no harm. On top of all the potential medical benefits, though, there is one positive factor I am completely at liberty to confirm and in my view made it worth it, and that was the effect on Derek's spirit, and how it drew him out in a way that lying in bed in his room, I felt, never could have.

Remember at this stage, as I say, he hadn't left the house, his safe place, especially his bed and bedroom. This was wonderful in one way as I obviously wanted him to feel safe and loved at home but I worried that he was retreating in an unhealthy way, that the outside world was becoming a distant, even hostile place to venture out into. This was something I knew we had to conquer.

So once arrangements were in place, I wanted to

make sure Derek understood this reasoning and the undertaking. It took me a couple of weeks to find the right moment to raise the subject. I needed to be sure that he understood, and by now I had learned to judge by the expression in his eyes when he was distracted, lost inside himself, and when he was able to focus on me. I waited until he used his good hand to buzz the alarm we'd installed, so I knew he was rested and he'd woken up.

'Darling,' I said, 'I've got something to ask you.'

In his eyes I saw a flicker of concern.

'Nothing bad,' I reassured him. 'In fact, something that could be really good. I've been doing some research and I've spoken to lots of people who've had a new type of treatment that they say can help speed up your healing.

'We know you're going to get there and we know that you're getting stronger every day,' I said, because I didn't want him to feel he had failed in any way with what we had done so far, or that this was a dramatic, desperate move born out of his lack of progress. In recent days, he had been crying a lot and saying that he'd let down the family and everyone who believed in him, which certainly wasn't what we felt – but said so much about his state of mind, even as he was doing us all proud with his determination and his fighting spirit.

'But I think this might be better and make things easier for you,' I added.

Before I could begin to explain further, he said. 'Yes, yes – do it!' in his staccato way. He was always missing out words that weren't vital to meaning, so personal pronouns like 'I' and 'you' went, adverbs like 'just' and 'also', and conjunctions like 'but' all disappeared. It was as if he only had enough energy to get out the essentials: 'yes', 'no', verbs and nouns.

'There's no guarantee, of course, because it is an experimental trial, but at the very least you would have a chance to be part of something that will help other people.'

I knew he would want this, because from the moment he'd regained consciousness he'd given approval for *any of his work* to be used for research and had already contributed to the growing body of knowledge about Covid – sadly because of things that hadn't been done in time, as opposed to positives that had helped him. But he communicated to me that he took comfort in that. I wanted him to realise that he could do something that would benefit himself and others – to make his story a tale of triumph, not of lessons learned from what went wrong. He is currently taking part in new trials for the NHS that won't benefit him – and he knows this – but he is still keen to participate.

'Yes, yes!' he said again.

'Okay, well, let me tell you what it involves, then,' I continued. 'We have to go abroad, which means travelling with an experienced nurse I've hired and flying, first to America and then on to Mexico, where you will get treatment.'

His eyes widened. 'How do that?'

I talked him through all my detailed planning: down to how we'd get him to the airport in an adapted vehicle and get him on the plane using a special lift.

'There will be people with you all the way,' I said.

He looked scared. 'Will *you* be with me?'

'Oh God, of course!' I said. 'I'm coming with you all the way. But it's a long flight, plus we will have to take things very slowly, so it will be more than 27 hours travelling in total. But we'll have lots of pauses and rests.

'We will have to get to the airport very early. I've arranged for you to have a room that you can lie flat in to recover from that bit of the journey. The airlines have been amazing and there will also be hospital support, both in the layover and when we get to Mexico, when we will be picked up in an ambulance and taken straight to the hospital.

'It will mean that we'll be on the plane at night probably, as that's the best way to make connections, but they've given us a special seat which reclines so you will be able to get flat or as flat as possible.'

We would have oxygen and all his food and supplies, and the nurse would be there in case anything went wrong. We also had a back-up plan ready if there were any dramas, but I didn't want to dwell too much on what could go wrong – I just wanted him to know enough to feel reassured.

'It's still a big thing, though, darling – what do you think about it?'

'And the kids – coming?'

'No, they can't come,' I said (thinking 'This is tough enough for me to deal with, let alone being responsible for them on such a trip too!'). 'They have school and also this way allows me to focus just on you ... *GMB* and Smooth have given me the leave to do it, but I don't want you to feel any pressure.'

'Who look after them?'

As all our time was spent caring for him and thinking about his needs, it was wonderful to hear him ask a question about them, about us. In fact, thinking about it, this was the first time he had expressed something so clear-sightedly, in such a 'dad way'. It almost made me cry.

'My mum and dad are going to come and stay; and your sister will be around when they're not. So it will be just you and me. Do you want to have time to think about it? Should I leave it with you to ponder?'

But there was something about his expression that told me he needed me to stay, so I just stayed quiet and sat back and let him stare at the ceiling as he thought about it.

A smile spread across his face as his eyes turned back to mine. 'Date night!'

I risked a joke and said, 'Yes, it will be – and possibly the mile high club as well, as our date will be in the air.'

I laughed as I said it.

It was Derek's stamp of approval – we were actually doing this.

The day came and Derek was awake before I needed to get him up. From the moment we got in the vehicle to head to the airport, I sensed a change in him. He was positioned upright in a special seat rather than his wheelchair, which immediately offered him more comfort, and his gaze when he looked out of the window had a new determination. It was very early in the morning, still dark, but his eyes stayed glued to the window, wanting to suck everything in.

I was on my phone for most of the journey, trying to sort out last-minute details. At one point, when I was talking to my lovely agent Matt, whose unwavering help with everything has gone far above and beyond his remit as agent, I lost my train of thought, and said, 'Oh God, hold on, hang on ...'

I wasn't aware that Derek was listening so intently, but after a while he said, 'Get on with it – Matt not got all day.'

Matt heard on the other end and started laughing, as did I, and it gave Matt the chance to say, 'That's the Derek I know and love!'

And Derek smiled.

When we pulled up at the airport, we had to contact

the medical team to come and help get us onto the plane. They were brilliant; their enthusiasm and expertise were truly remarkable.

I could tell Derek was anxious because of the logistical challenges ahead, which would involve considerable discomfort for him.

I asked if he was all right. 'Quiet. Concentrating,' he said.

'Fair enough,' I thought.

It felt like an entirely reasonable response bearing in mind how strange the situation was – the strangest we've ever been in, probably. He knew I understood and we were experiencing a depth of communication and understanding which was wonderful. It's difficult to describe how peculiar and surreal the situation was, and yet still we were communicating in a profound conversation, with very few words. Despite the challenges that lay before us, the bond between us felt reassuringly intact, reinforcing the depth of our connection as we set out to traverse uncharted territory together.

In that moment, a surge of love for him flowed through me and enveloped my being. And hope too, weaving in and out like a magical ribbon. It felt like one of those guided visualisations for de-stressing or self-expression, but it was in three-dimensional, sensational techni-colour – and it was real and tangible. Love and hope, the strongest cocktail on earth.

We had to be at the airport five hours before takeoff

because there were so many procedures to go through. All the equipment, medical supplies and liquid food had to be security checked as they would for any other passenger. We also had no way of knowing how Derek would cope with all this movement and travelling, so we had to build in rest times, when he could be transferred to medical areas to rest. We also had to do last-minute pad changes, feeds, meds and checks, so getting him onto the plane was a huge challenge. He had to be lifted up in a special airline lift before anybody else came aboard and positioned in his seat. But once on board, he relaxed; it was amazing.

We had seats next to each other, obviously; I could see his eyes all the time and he smiled, and I squeezed his hand. He's always been nervous of flying, so I wondered how on earth he was going to feel now. He'd only learned to deal with his fear because he wanted to put on a brave face for the kids so they didn't get scared; but after all that he'd been through, surely this was going to freak him out?

He coped remarkably well and then exhaustion took over, and he fell asleep. But only for about ten minutes and he woke up when the stewardess passed. She asked him how he was and he smiled. It must've been wonderful for him to be out seeing people, experiencing some sort of normality ... that felt healing in itself. I managed to set up the TV so he was propped up enough to see it and we chose a film together. I read out the list and he picked *The Bridges of Madison County*. I watched it too, not having seen it in years, and blubbed my eyes out at various points and looked across to see he was blubbing too. It really did feel like a date night. The first time for a long while that we felt we were in a marriage, not a caring partnership between nurse and patient.

At the end of the treatment, Derek had further tests and all the specialists there felt that they could already see improvements, but this was only the first of at least four stages that would span at least two years so we had a long way to go. As we headed back to the airport, though, to fly home, I sensed that just being told something positive by a doctor, after hearing so many negatives and having so many setbacks, was a balm in itself.

However, our journey wasn't over. We had to repeat the arduous process of navigating through the airport, with all our contraptions and challenges. This particular airport was not so used to dealing with sick people as the UK one, and there was the language barrier which meant lots of shouting and hand-waving from concerned staff. I noticed a hint of distress on his face, but when I asked him, he gave me a dismissive glance to brush it off. I could tell he was mustering all his concentration and strength, trying to be resilient. I purposely held back as the crane lifted him up, with me standing on the platform behind him.

When we reached the level of the plane's door, he started gesturing wildly with his right hand. The workers were perplexed, looking at me with concern. I craned my neck, trying to catch a glimpse of Derek's expression. He repeated the gesture, and suddenly it hit me like a ton of bricks. He wanted to touch the side of the plane – a ritual he had developed to overcome his fear of flying. Every time we boarded a plane, he would tap three times and say, 'Loving you, Mr Plane. Make sure you carry us safely there, won't you?' The kids had grown fond of this little tradition, and they too would participate. It had become our family's good luck charm.

Amid all the chaos and stress, I couldn't believe that he had focused on this ritual. Somewhere deep inside, he'd found the strength to take control and connect with a playful, mischievous part of himself. Regardless of what the medical scans revealed, this gesture felt like a breakthrough. I did my best to explain in my broken Spanish that he wanted the crane to shift him slightly to the right. The workers looked puzzled, but they complied. He reached out, tapped three times, and whispered, 'Keep us safe, Mr Plane.' He turned to me, a smile illuminating his face, before tears streamed down his cheeks.

I embraced him tightly, overcome by the magnitude of the moment. In the same instant, I realised we were in danger of delaying the entire flight. 'Let's get on board,' I urged, giving his hand a final squeeze. Once we were settled in our seats, I couldn't help but feel that this was the beginning of a whole new chapter – a chapter filled with resilience, hope, and the unwavering love that had carried us through it all.

Chapter 8

Reaching for the Strawberry

In some ways Derek's physical health was like a giant game of whack-a-mole – every time we got on top of one problem, another, potentially even more deadly one, cropped up where we least expected it. But unravelling his mind, finding out what he was thinking, who he was now and how we could relate to it, was more like a game of Cluedo.

Without speech, without the usual expressions to signal what he thought and wanted, we had to be a bit like detectives, but instead of Miss Scarlett in the dining room with the lead piping, it was a case of Derek in his bed, needing, what? A pad change? Some nutrition? Some company?

As much as we were struggling with the way Covid inflammation had affected Derek's brain, it was even more of a challenge for the expert 'brain detectives' whose care he was under – the neurologists and neuro-psychologists – because he presented in such a different way from other brain injuries they had investigated. When they gave him tests to try to assess his cognition, his responses were so varied and unpredictable that he confounded them every time.

They usually began with simple cognitive tests, like asking him his name and date of birth and seeing if he could point at the calendar to show us what date he thought it might be, encouraging him to say it out loud as well. Even now, more than three years on, he still can't work out what the day or month is, despite the hints we give him and despite the riot of spring blossom or autumn leaves outside his window, and not even when he has been told the date or month just an hour earlier.

When I was with him during these sessions with the neuropsychologists, I would sometimes try to help. I remember asking him, 'When is my birthday?'

'May 4th,' he answered straight away.

Then I asked, 'When was my birthday?'

'A week ago, maybe?' he said.

'Okay, so what month is it now?' I asked.

'I don't know,' he replied, and burst into tears.

The lack of connection was confounding – and I could see it confounded Derek, too.

In another session, one of the neuropsychologists asked him to name five farmyard animals. When he couldn't do it, it made him cry. To distract him, the neuropsychologist picked up a Father's Day card from Darcey, which was still next to his bed. In her card, Darcey had referred to a standing joke they've always had, about the prefrontal cortex of the brain. Admittedly, this is not what dads and daughters usually joke about, but I guess that's what you get with a psychologist dad! And Darcey loved it. Whenever Darcey had pushed too hard for something that Derek thought was seriously unwise, foolish or even potentially dangerous, they had always had some banter about it, and he would say, 'No, Darcey', again and again. Then, if she continued to push, he'd say, 'I know you think you are right, but in this case you are wrong. And I know why you are wrong, and you don't. At your age, the prefrontal cortex in your brain isn't fully formed, so you don't know about these dangers.'

It was brilliant; she couldn't argue because she knew he understood psychology and the development of the brain. She would be incandescent with fury but rendered almost speechless, left to mutter 'You wait till I get older', before letting him give her a massive hug. It was their thing – he'd never tried this argument with Billy because he knew she secretly loved the battle and that he wouldn't.

I was very moved when, without any prompting from me, she wrote in the card, 'I am so proud of you, Dad. You are my total hero. But you had better get better quickly because every day I am getting older and my prefrontal cortex is getting more formed and soon you will never be able to win an argument.'

She told me that she had done it to motivate him.

'Do you think he will get it?' I asked, wondering if he would even remember their joke.

'Hopefully,' she said.

He read it and burst into tears, and then he hugged her tightly. I cried too, because of course the brutal irony was that Covid had now most likely affected *his* prefrontal cortex.

'You are cleverer than me, Darcey. But still your dad,' he said.

He insisted that Darcey's card stayed next to his bed at all times and it remains there to this day.

When the neuropsychologist read the card, it was clear he was a bit shocked, and it certainly did seem like fairly black humour from a teenager to a father in Derek's position!

'Did she really write this?' he asked.

'Yes,' Derek replied, chuckling.

The neuropsychologist raised his eyebrows. 'And did you really say that to her?!!'

'Yes, I did,' Derek said.

'What did she say? How did she react?' he asked.

Derek laughed. 'Furious, absolutely furious.'

The neuropsychologist, sensing an opportunity to draw out the conversation, pushed on and got Derek to explain what he meant by prefrontal cortex in teenagers. And he did – it was a very staccato conversation, but he used all the right terms and gave precisely the right explanation.

On another occasion, the neuropsychologist brought along some books about Italian art and talked to Derek about the pictures he loved, using the books as a prop to spark a conversation. He asked Derek if he'd been to Italy, where he'd been and if he liked art; he also shared his own likes and dislikes with him.

Derek was wide-eyed but could only answer 'yes' or 'no', and sometimes, 'I don't know.'

The neuropsychologist left it at that and then didn't see Derek for three weeks. When he came back to see him, he started setting up his computer to take notes and, almost rhetorically, half to himself, said, 'Now where were we? What were we talking about last time?'

Without even looking at him, Derek answered straight away, 'Italy – you loved Tuscany, weren't keen on Botticelli.'

The neuropsychologist nearly fell off his chair.

He called me straight after the session. 'He remembered, even when *I* had forgotten – I couldn't believe it! Yet then when I asked him to name ten colours, he couldn't – it's so bizarre.'

Well, if he was bewildered, imagine how challenged we felt. But love made it a challenge that we relished.

The kids were brilliant with Derek, albeit in very

different ways. Billy seemed to intuitively know how to lift his dad's spirits and make him laugh, and Darcey was always quietly watching him to check his breathing was okay or that he was safely swallowing his food; whether or not he was in pain or needed a hydrating sip of water. She was always looking for clues and often saw them before I did, or he did. She constantly asked him questions, which weren't simply about trying to glean the little practicalities of what he needed but finding out what he was thinking and feeling. And she was always trying to show him that she was on his side, that she 'got him': how he was now and how he could relate to us; how he could feel our love and be part of our family. At the same time, we didn't want him to feel interrogated, knowing there was a balance to be struck between stimulation and ensuring the loving relationships in his life felt as they always had. He wanted her to be his daughter – and me his wife – rather than his carer.

Sometimes, when we pushed too hard, he put his hand out and grimaced. That was when he had zero words; then, later, he'd say, 'Don't put me on the spot.'

I learned to ask one question at a time and then wait for him to answer while the seconds seemed to stretch on interminably. If I asked more than one question at a time, even if it was essentially asking the same thing such as, 'Do you want a blanket, or would that be too heavy, or maybe if I put the fire on …?' To me it seemed like I was asking one question: are you warm enough? But I learned that, because of the way his brain was relearning how to process information and how hard it was for him to retrieve the answers, to him it felt like a barrage because he had to consciously stop and think about each one.

I realised early on that so much of his time had been spent in a hospital bed that he desperately needed sensory stimulation. I decided to start small, with cues from the natural world, and took leaves into the hospital and got him to touch and feel and sniff them. Later, I picked flowers from the garden and brought them into his room at home. I could see that being stuck in a box for so long – in various hospitals – had saved him physically, but hadn't helped him mentally, and I knew it would be vital to his recovery to get him outside as much as possible when he was strong enough. We installed a lift in the house to make it easier to get him into our back garden. (There's no direct access from the back door because we live on a hill and you have to go down some steps.)

Maddeningly, the lift kept breaking down and every time it stopped working it was weeks before we could get the company to come back to repair it. But, as luck would have it, I had to do some filming for a gardening show at home and one day there was a team of directors and camera people in the garden, so I thought, 'Right, this is my moment to get Derek outside.'

Together we carried him down the steps in his wheel-chair. The carers were nervous about it and it was definitely not recommended, because of course there was a risk he might slip in the chair on the way down and hurt himself. I felt confident that we had enough people to do it safely and that it was worth it so that he could get some fresh air and be outside in nature. 'I'll take the risk,' I reassured the carers. 'I'll put it on your record in case anything goes wrong.' Thankfully nothing did.

Once in the garden, Derek looked around, a bit wide-eyed, but seemed renewed by it. It was autumn and the boughs of the apple trees were bending with the weight of ripening fruit. 'Fancy picking an apple?' I asked Derek, and he actually reached up, grasped an apple and pulled it off the branch!

It was an unbelievable breakthrough. He'd wanted something and he'd reached for it. Yes, I had prompted him to do it but I hadn't had to tell him *how* to do it, with specific instructions such as: lift up your arm, stretch out your hand, clasp the apple.

On another occasion, after our trip to Mexico, I wheeled him out into the front garden, thinking I could take his socks off and lift his legs so he could put his feet on the grass. Again, the carers weren't sure but I was more confident, having undertaken a long journey with him, and felt it was important for him to be outside as much as possible. He hadn't felt the earth beneath his feet since March 2020 and I hoped it would ground him, as he had always loved walking about barefoot before. He seemed to enjoy feeling the grass between his toes, but within minutes it became too much – sensory overload, probably. We always had to take things so gently.

We were doing everything we could think of to bring him out and back into the world, into our world.

'Dad loves sandalwood,' the kids said.

We found a small oil burner in his study and the kids bought some essence of sandalwood with their pocket money.

'Do you like it, Dad?' they asked, as its familiar scent filled the air.

He smiled.

Hoping that our love could provide a form of therapy for him, we played board games together, ones that we knew challenged his recall – dominoes and memory games where you put cards on the table, turn them over and try to remember where they are. The kids were really patient when Derek couldn't do it and tried to make it seem as though they were struggling, too. It was wonderful to watch, but after a while Derek sensed they were accommodating him and didn't want to continue. Being reminded of his limitations seemed to send him crashing into a wall of frustration and despondency.

Speaking of frustration ... bizarrely, he liked playing the game Frustration. You'd think it would be something that would make him even more frustrated! But moving the counters along the spaces was therapy for Derek –

even the action of reaching out and pressing the button to roll the dice was a useful challenge – and it was a game he'd often played with the kids when they were much younger, so they loved playing it, too. When they'd played it before Covid, Derek had made it really fun for Darcey and Bill by inventing phrases for moments in the game: when someone surged into the lead, say, or fell behind, or won. These phrases entered our family language to the extent that the kids thought they were stock phrases people used when playing any kind of game. Darcey told Derek that she and Bill had been surprised to find that other families didn't use them. It was another reminder of Derek's love of words and how his mastery of language had always defined and bound our family together.

Playing games seemed to bring his old self back, but there was poignancy in it too, because it became wearing for the children as the weeks turned into months and then years. It's hard to keep taking the same joy in the same things, hard to keep the intensity of love and emotion going. I sensed that Derek also felt this; the excitement of being home wasn't enough as time stretched on. Playing games together had been so rewarding the first, second, third and even the twentieth time, but what we wanted to feel was that we were on a ladder climbing higher and higher, rather than negotiating stepping stones across a bog, unable to see where to jump to next, through the thick fog. And I was conscious that I didn't want to use the kids as therapists for Derek in this way. They had their own issues and sometimes needed simply to be kids.

One issue that baffled us was why his voice was so quiet and his specialist needed to further investigate the reasons for this. Was it purely neurological, something to do with the connections between the brain and the voice box? Or was it physical – had his vocal cords been damaged? While we were waiting for these referrals to come up, a speech therapist advised us that we could help increase the volume of Derek's voice by putting a decibel meter next to us and encouraging him to hit a certain level on it. The idea was that every time he didn't hit that level, we should ignore him and carry on talking. We could hear that he was trying and sometimes he did hit the required level, but at other times fatigue overwhelmed him and he just gave up, retreated and stayed silent.

I decided that communication was more important than volume because, if trying to get him to speak louder was in fact exhausting him and making him less likely to attempt to communicate, it would create more problems than it would solve. It was also turning family time into a therapy session, when so much of his life was already a painful struggle. It was such a fine balance between us helping him and adding to the frustration of his life – and I didn't want him to feel he was being tested at times when he should just be feeling loved, supported and understood.

We also wanted to feel that he understood us – I particularly craved this because I felt that Derek had always been the person who 'got' me the most. Sometimes I'd make a joke and he would laugh and other times he simply wouldn't react. We wondered why he responded in this way. Was it because his brain couldn't cope with it cognitively? Was it because he couldn't find *anything* funny just then, or because he didn't find that particular joke funny? (Entirely possible with my jokes!) Was it a rejection of me or a rejection in that moment, of everything but the pain and the confusion inside his head? Obviously, on one level, I didn't care whether he laughed at a joke or not but on another level it felt as though I constantly had to steel myself not to feel hurt if he didn't respond. I hated it when it happened with the kids, who were riding this emotional rollercoaster as well.

Before he came home in April 2021, I remember warning the kids: 'Daddy is going to be changed. He's still very weak: he can't move and can't really speak, but he does understand more than you think. We will have to take care of him.'

Of course, two solemn pairs of eyes looked at me sadly. 'We will definitely do that. We'd love to do that.' Then, after a pause, Billy hesitantly said, 'Mum, will he be able to speak eventually?'

'Well, we hope so, when he's stronger, but we just don't know.'

'Cos that's all I really want, Mum. I don't mind if he's

in a wheelchair – that's no problem at all. I just want him to be Dad and laugh and joke and talk. Then everything can be, you know, normal. It won't feel like we've lost him.'

When he first came home, the kids were so full of joy at his mere presence, such was their love for him. It was as if you could see their hearts bursting out of them. Every evening they would rush in from school, desperate to see their dad. Having him there, being able to hug and squeeze him, was easily enough for them during those first weeks and months. The days when he could manage a smile or a nod or even a 'well done' when they gave him a bit of news were exhilarating for all of us. But for each time he did this, there were so many days when he couldn't react at all; so for every heart-lifting moment there was also a heartbreaking one.

Billy got back from school one day with a big bit of news. 'I did well in my maths test!' This was huge to him as he referred to maths as his 'worst enemy'. Derek had spent so much time building Billy's confidence with maths and I knew that, yes, he was pleased to tell me but it was really Derek he wanted to celebrate with. But Derek could only smile passively. Billy was crushed. He went out into the hall and I said to him, 'It's not Dad's fault, he can't do it right now.'

'I know, don't go on about it,' Bill replied. I desperately wanted to keep the closeness between them and it hurt me to see *him* disappointed, but I found my attempts to make excuses or smooth things over were actually making it worse, so I had to take a step back.

As much as I tried to do research and keep on top of what might be the cause of some of Derek's physical challenges, which I figured would help me head them off at the pass, I accepted that we were in the hands of the brilliant health teams and carers – and, I guess, waiting for medical science generally to catch up with Covid. But in terms of his spirit, his mind, surely those who loved him – his family and friends – were the real experts? After all, a huge part of the reason why the specialists released him into our care in the first place on 21st April, 2021, was so that he could be stimulated by us – fired by our love for him, and his love for us.

But now his spirit appeared to be declining. I had known for some time that, at the very least, he was going to be in trauma and shock. In Italy, there were cases of Covid patients who'd spent a long time in a coma and intensive care and had experienced a version of post-traumatic stress disorder. This could lead to all sorts of symptoms, including intrusive memories, nightmares, insomnia, anxiety and feeling numb or detached – and any of these could prevent Derek from 'coming back to us' in the full sense, in his spirit and in his Derek-ness.

And, of course, that's what the kids and I wanted: amid all the fear and anxiety about his physical health and the challenges of caring for him, what we really feared was that we'd lost him – the essence of him, whatever that might be. We longed to have him back, his personality intact. Our love embraced who he was now and validated who he'd been before, and it was vital for his spirit that he felt seen and understood in both incarnations.

There were also times, though, when he actively tried to make me laugh. He'd taken to watching the same films over and over again – usually Elton John's *Rocketman*, *Hamilton* or *Billy Elliot* – and he'd cry at the same points, laugh at the same points and repeat words of dialogue out loud. He took comfort in the familiarity of the films but was also aware of the repetitive nature of rewatching them endlessly. I would often watch them with him and as we approached certain moments, he'd always make the same joke – but he was aware that he was making the same joke. I'd say, 'Oh my God, you're going to make the same joke again, aren't you? Don't do it, don't do it!' He would start laughing – knowing it was coming up – and then, barely able to get the words out because he knew he was repeating it and was laughing so much, he would say it again. The first time it happened it was exhilarating. It was him trying to reach out to me to bond. And as we looked at each other, I could feel the connection and love between us. I treasured it and he never tired of it. There was comfort in it for him.

While we had fun watching the same films multiple times, I was still keen to draw him out.

As I was racking my brain for ideas, a jokey article in

a magazine gave me a breakthrough. The headline was, 'Why being nosy and FOMO is a cure for pain', and it was intriguing. It turned out that a research study at the University of Melbourne had given a group of people a piece of kit to place on their leg that would heat up and eventually get painfully hot. When this was done in isolation, people taking part instantly pulled the hot plate off, but if they were given a game to play while wearing it with the chance to get bits of gossip about the other players or some news, they were able to bear the pain. And they were prepared to hang on as the pain increased *and* increased to get even more news. A lightbulb went on in my head. Curiosity, curiosity! I couldn't believe I hadn't thought of it before.

Let me explain: when I finished *I'm a Celebrity* and came back from the jungle at the beginning of January 2020, Derek and I began writing a book together. It was going to be called *The Naked Power of Curiosity*. I had a theory that curiosity is really powerful and Derek was compiling the psychological research to back it up. One study that really interested him showed that people with depression and serious mental health issues exhibited little or no curiosity and asked very few questions. He was fascinated because one of the things he loved about me was that I was always curious and kept asking why. He called me the ultimate chitter-chatterer, although it did drive him mad that I would talk to absolutely anyone (people on trains and buses are particular victims!) and always wanted to know about their lives and what they got up to.

'Why do you need to know?' he'd ask. 'You're never going to see that person again.'

'I love it!' I would respond. 'I always learn something from talking to people, even if it's just a little thing that gets me thinking and leads me onto something else ...'

'You are a fruit loop,' he would say affectionately. 'You really are "Curiosity Kate".'

Obviously we never got to finish the book we were writing. We barely even began. Maybe one day we will.

I remember relating to Derek a story that I thought justified my curiosity and my obsession with why it was so powerful for living life to the full.

This Zen tale has been told for centuries in China and still sends a shiver down my spine every time I hear it. It was first told to me by a location director on the set of *The Bourne Supremacy*, which I visited to interview Matt Damon and Julia Stiles for the American entertainment show, *Access Hollywood*. That particular part of the movie was set in Berlin and we were filming in a very bleak part of the city on a freezing cold day in February. As always on film sets, there was a lot of hanging around and precious little shelter to do the hanging around in. As I hugged my steaming cup of tea, the woman who had been charged with looking after me said, 'Are you okay? I am sure we'll get a chance to get you in with Matt and Julia soon.'

'Don't worry,' I replied, 'this is great, so much to see and learn.' And while I didn't say this bit out loud, I was thinking that I had my curiosity to keep me warm.

The second director picked up on this and said, 'Oh, I remember when just being here was so thrilling – it's good to have people like you around to remind us of how great days like this really are.' We then went on to talk about staying interested and engaged with what you do, and he told me this story:

A monk is taking a walk just outside the monastery walls when a huge tiger suddenly leaps out of the bushes. He is momentarily shocked, but a second later starts to run. A few seconds after that, with the tiger catching up, he reaches a cliff with a long drop and huge rocks below. He has to decide what to do and does the only thing he can think of – he quickly scrambles over the edge and hangs by his fingertips from the cliff top.

Above him crouches a snarling, drooling tiger. Hundreds of feet below lie jagged rocks and crashing waves. He hangs on for as long as he can. And just when he thinks he can hang on no longer and will have to let go and crash onto the rocks, he sees something out of the corner of his eye. A flash of red. He looks and the red disappears. Then again a flash of red. Now he no longer notices the hot breath of the tiger or its saliva dripping down on his face. He doesn't even hear the deafening noise of the waves smashing on the rocks below. His mind is totally focused on the flash of red.

What can it be? Why is it there? How can he get to it?

His thoughts compel him to try to reach it. With his last ounce of strength, he stretches towards it and, inch by painful inch, manages to ease himself close enough to grab it. It's a strawberry. It looks so good. He reaches out, nearly falling off the cliff edge, plucks it and places it in his mouth. He eats it and it's the juiciest, most delicious strawberry he has ever tasted.

So here is the question: what is the tiger, what are the rocks below and what indeed is the strawberry? What do they symbolise?

I believe the tiger represents Time, constantly breathing down our necks; the sea is all the challenges of Life that set us back and distract us from truly living before the ultimate challenge, Death, which no one can avoid, and is always there, waiting to swallow us up. So we have to make the most of everything in between. Unless we let our Curiosity spur us on to reach for the strawberry of Life, we will never taste its sweetness and our efforts just to hold on – just to survive, not thrive will have been pointless. What's more, while Curiosity helps us reach for Life, we don't notice the ticking of Time or the certainty of Death; in that moment we forget the challenges and struggles that haunt us.

This is the memory that popped into my head as I had my lightbulb moment. 'Oh my God,' I said, literally jumping out of my seat and shocking the kids in the process. 'We need to reach for the strawberry!'

There was always going to be something that went wrong, always something that set Derek back and maybe we could never entirely fix the situation, so we had to reconnect him with his innate curiosity and excite him about his life.

'Right,' I thought, 'we'll have to take matters into our own hands and somehow find the strawberry for him to metaphorically reach for.' We needed something to stimulate Derek and we needed to make new memories for us as a family.

We had to get him out of that bed and out of the house. And so we decided to push the boundaries, to create memories that would fire his senses and ignite our entire family.

I felt that music might be the way because he always reacted so positively to it. On one occasion when he was in hospital there was a group of volunteers who went round the wards, reading to the patients and also encouraging them to sing. This was part of a programme to lift patients' morale, but also studies have found that words are often more accessible to people with diminished communication when they sing, because singing and speech are controlled by different parts of the brain.

On this occasion, Derek was unable to say much to the visitor, so she suggested singing and gave him a choice of tunes. Derek picked 'Country Roads' and she was blown away that he was word-perfect and sang it all the way through. She asked him if she could film it on his iPad and then the nurses sent it to me on my phone. I didn't even realise that he knew that song particularly well, but it was very poignant because he was looking straight into the camera lens, singing 'Country roads, take me home', almost pleading with me to listen to his lament. It was utterly heartbreaking, but also spellbinding to see how the words came.

We'd played music to Derek too, when he was in his coma and also as he started to emerge. Sir Elton John had got in touch when Derek was first sick to try and help – at the time he, too, had a close friend in intensive care with Covid. He was very moved when I said that I was playing his music to Derek. As Derek got stronger and came home, Elton said he would love to have the chance to meet Derek one day and love him to attend one of his concerts once Covid restrictions lifted and he could get back on the road. It seemed as if it might never happen because every time a date near to where we lived was scheduled, Derek had a setback. The January dates in London, where we live, at the start of 2023 seemed like our last shot.

Elton was performing at the legendary O2 in London. We knew we had to make it happen, to do something extraordinary that would connect Derek's emotional past with a blazing moment in the present. I wanted to go for myself and the kids too, but I knew it would be especially wonderful for Derek. It was an emotional step we had to take, a way to make him a part of something incredible in the present, rather than constantly looking back to the past.

We got in touch with Elton's extraordinary crew and the amazing disability team at the O2, but it wasn't going to be a walk in the park. We needed extra carers by Derek's side because we were venturing into uncharted territory. We worked with a transport company's mobility team to ensure the set-up was just right, taking into account Derek's constant back pain and his existing nerve concerns. Sitting in a wheelchair for anything longer than 20 minutes was very uncomfortable for him.

On the morning of the concert, Derek seemed so weak I feared we would have to cancel but he was determined to go. As soon as he woke up, he remembered what was happening and asked me if we were still going. I assured him that, if he felt up to it, we would make it happen. And we did.

I made sure I was dressed up for the occasion, sporting an Elton-esque top and shiny gold boots that I knew he would approve of, if only he could see them. Derek had on one of his favourite shirts from the old days, rather than a hospital gown or the plain, comfortable T-shirts he had grown accustomed to, and he looked more like himself than he had in a long time. The kids were also dressed up to the nines.

The journey to the O2 was nerve-racking. Every bump on the road seemed to resonate through Derek's body and

I felt every jolt along with him. But the incredible thing was the sheer excitement radiating between him and the kids. Darcey and Billy were buzzing with anticipation, and they had even brought Cadbury's Éclair sweets, which are Derek's favourites and had always been a staple on family trips. We shared them on the journey, laughing and savouring the moment. And then Derek, unprompted, suggested playing some Elton John music to get us in the mood. It was his own idea, that made the kids squeal with delight. In that instant, Derek took the lead and breathed life into our adventure.

As we approached the O2, staff guided us around the back of the arena and into the backstage area. The energy was palpable, as it was for everybody attending that night. It was a particularly monumental occasion for our family and our excitement was infectious. Even the driver became emotional. 'I feel like this is something amazing, I'm proud to be part of it,' he said, almost on the verge of tears.

I had worried that once we stepped inside the O2, it would be overwhelming for Derek. Bright lights, loud noises and the vastness of the venue could be overwhelming for anyone. As we emerged into the disabled area and onto the viewing platform, specifically designed to accommodate wheelchair users, my worries eased. The scale of the arena, filled with thousands and thousands of excited people, was mind-blowing. I wondered what it was doing to Derek, but his wide-eyed expression didn't convey fear. It was as if he was being energised, accelerated in some way.

'Are you okay?' I asked him, concerned. 'Do you want your ear defenders on?'

After a brief pause, he blurted out, 'No. Want to hear.'

And then it began. Needless to say, it was beyond wonderful. It was Elton. The music resonated with every single person in the auditorium, taking us back to different eras in our lives. And for Derek it was even more profound, connecting him to the moments when he had been coming out of the coma, listening to Elton's songs. It felt as if he had burst out of a bubble, like Truman in *The Truman Show*, and emerged before us. Maybe I was the only one who could see it, as the changes in his expressions were subtle, but I knew deep down that he was truly present.

People from all around came up to us, saying how good it was to see Derek there. He was visibly moved. I had told him countless times about the messages from strangers, the people who approached me on the street to ask about him, but now he could truly feel it. He was there, a part of it all, immersed in the incredible love and support from the kids, the carers and all the Elton fans around us. Strangers shared their stories with us, recounting the challenges they had faced and the loved ones they had lost. It was overwhelming, but in the most marvellous way.

The power of music to touch us all, to create

connections and stir emotions, was on full display that night. And in that sea of people, Derek was no longer just a patient or a person with limitations. He was Derek, a symbol of strength and resilience, embraced by the love and camaraderie of those around us. It was a night that will be forever etched in our hearts.

The concert was long – Elton knows how to give his fans their money's worth! And I was concerned that Derek hadn't been out of bed, sitting upright, for this long since Covid had first gripped him. Of course, for everybody else, they didn't want it to end! As the night wore on, I noticed Derek's posture deteriorating. He was slumping more and more, but his gaze remained fixed on the stage. I suggested the ear defenders again, hoping they would help reduce the overwhelming sensory stimulation.

'Maybe,' he said. 'Wait, though.'

He started to shake, which is what he sometimes did when his energy had gone, and then went very floppy. The carers were concerned and I thought, 'Maybe this is it, maybe we're going to have to go.'

I asked Derek, 'Do we need to go?'

He and I both looked at the children, absolutely loving it. I could tell Derek didn't want to ruin it for them, but I didn't want him to leave by himself. 'Why don't we step outside for a bit?' I suggested. 'I'll ask if we can find somewhere flat to lie down and you can just regroup a bit, reboot.'

'Okay.'

We wheeled him outside and I tried to find somewhere for him to lie down. The corridors were quite busy at the O2 and a lot of people had clearly been celebrating with a pint or two. I tried to protect Derek, not that anyone was going to do him any harm, it was just a bit loud and raucous, but it suddenly must have felt very overwhelming for somebody who had been in isolation for so long. It wasn't obvious where he could lie down, so a carer and I found a large disabled toilet and, inspired by the twin spirits of necessity and invention, managed get him into an almost flat position using the nappy changer and the frame that we'd brought with us to help manoeuvre him.

We turned the lights out and stayed really quiet, creating a little oasis of calm. We also gave him some water through his PEG and some liquid nutrition to give him a boost of energy and sugar. After a while he seemed to revive and said, 'What now?'

I said, 'It's up to you. We can either go home now or we can go back for the end as I don't think there's much left.'

'Want to go back,' he said.

We carefully wove our way back into the auditorium, found our place and were settling down as Elton began speaking. He was thanking people who had helped him through his life and wanted to dedicate his performance to them. He mentioned Lulu, who was there that night, and he talked about Bernie Taupin, his lyricist, and what their incredible partnership meant to him. He also thanked his bandmaster, who had supported him all the way through the early days in LA, and he thanked those in the band too.

And then, unbelievably, he said, 'The people that I'm really thrilled are here, because they've been through hell over the last few years, are Kate Garraway and Derek Draper and their kids. They've inspired me, I'm sure they've inspired you. They've never given up and I'm so thrilled they are here. To say that they've been through a lot is an understatement of huge proportions and I want to dedicate this song to the people I mentioned before, but especially to you guys.'

Then the first notes of 'Don't Let the Sun Go Down On Me' started up. Derek was in tears. The kids were in tears, I was in tears and so were the carers who were with us and the people all around us. They were standing up, clapping, waving, smiling, blowing kisses and saying, 'Well done!', but also respectfully keeping back, realising that this was an intense moment, just for us.

It was the strawberry to end all strawberries!!!

Just as remarkable in a different way was what happened afterwards on the journey home.

Derek was exhausted. And yet strangely still so awake and present. Earlier, we had wondered if he'd be able to get out of bed at all, and now here we were, nearly 11 hours later, and he was still wide awake.

There's always a long queue as you drive away from

the O2. As we slowly moved through the traffic, Derek suddenly spoke to the driver.

'Why don't you take that road?'

The driver said, 'I would, but there are roadworks.'

I couldn't believe Derek had remembered a different route. Our carer, Jake, said it was like a miracle. And then Derek turned to the kids and said, 'Do you want to go to Legoland tomorrow?'

Again, I couldn't believe what I was hearing. He'd come up with a suggestion for something he knew they'd love to do, something that was not even in the context of where we were. This may seem small but he had not done this kind of thinking since Covid. The kids were delighted and concerned. 'Don't you think you'll be tired, Dad?'

'Maybe,' he said, 'but isn't it about time we did something like that?'

Bill said, 'But you don't even like theme parks, Dad.'

'Want to do it with you,' he replied.

Of course, in the end, he was completely wiped out for the next few days. His fatigue was beyond belief and he wasn't even able to get out of bed. Bill kept saying to him, 'We will go to Legoland, Dad, I promise.'

We'd had that moment, we'd reached for that strawberry. When I relayed the evening to Sir Elton, he said, 'Well, that's what it's all about for me, it makes everything worthwhile.' I resolved to find more opportunities to stimulate him and bring us all together.

Even if we never got the chance to do anything like this again, we'd experienced a moment of joy that wasn't just about the past, it was alive in the here and now and I knew that it had boosted his spirit immeasurably. When it comes down to it, what is anyone's life but just a collection of wonderful moments that make you feel fulfilled?

The last thing he said before he went to bed was, 'I won't let the sun go down on me.'

We were never going to let the sun go down on him, not without a fight. We'd got this far, we weren't stopping now. Little did I know, though, that I had a battle with myself and my own spirit on the horizon.

Chapter 9

The Dark Side

Friday has always been my favourite day of the week. It's the Christmas Eve of weekdays, isn't it? Perhaps this Friday feeling has its roots in childhood: the buzz of expectation and exhilaration when the school bell rang at the end of the day; the racing home and the relief as you dumped your scratchy uniform in the laundry bin (or on the floor!) and put on something comfy, relishing the expanse of the weekend ahead.

Derek loved Fridays too. We had always tried to avoid making plans for Friday nights – or at least made plans to do nothing apart from just being with each other and unwinding from the week, sharing updates and little moans, simply indulging in the joy of being together.

This particular Friday felt especially good because it had been a great week. That day's *GMB* had gone really well – ratings were on the up and there was a real Friday vibe among the crew.

Even better, no emergencies had arisen to drive Derek back into hospital and all his medical appointments had seemed promising: new specialists were offering opportunities to test things that hadn't been looked at yet; new referrals had been booked in and there was even the prospect of Derek going into a new trial. And I'd not had any panicky calls from carers that morning. The district nurse had been in touch, but only to let me know that the infection around Derek's feeding tube entry point was receding and that his blood pressure was relatively good.

Also, Derek's carer Jake had sent a video for me to watch while I was on air at Smooth Radio of Derek doing some of the arm exercises we had been working on. Jake texted, 'Derek wanted me to show you because he's proud he's doing so well. He wanted you to see.' Derek was smiling into the camera. 'God, I love him,' I thought, as I looked at his eyes, staring hard into the phone camera lens, letting me know he was fighting, sharing his triumphs with me. 'Oh and he's got a new favourite film: *Life of Brian* – *he* actually asked me for it!' Jake added. Any time that Derek initiated a thought, rather than having it suggested to him, was like opening champagne. It meant he had been able to think of something and find a way of asking for it.

I am always keen to get home before the kids get back

from school on a Friday so, after my show, I jumped on the back of a taxi motorbike to get me home quicker. The air felt warm as we wove our way through the traffic jams and I felt relaxed enough to give my friend Vickie a quick call. I'd been meaning to call her for weeks but I'd been flat-out and hadn't had a second to do anything other than send her a quick text message update on how things were going. She didn't answer, so I left a message: 'Hi babe, hope you're all good. We actually had a rather lovely week in the Draper household and I don't want to tempt fate but you've got to celebrate the good things when you can, haven't you? Hope you've got a lovely weekend planned and let's catch up.'

When I got home, I hopped off the bike and checked my watch. Great – I had time to do a handover with the carer, chuck a load of washing on *and* spend a bit of time with Derek before the kids got back.

I quietly opened the door to Derek's room, in case he was asleep – and there he was, my husband, watching *Life of Brian*. At least, he looked like my husband; he had the same thick brown hair and heavy-lidded dark brown eyes. His left hand was resting on his knee as he lay in bed; his wedding ring wasn't as shiny as it was on our wedding day, when we walked down the aisle of St Mary's in Primrose Hill, beaming with happiness – but he was fiddling with the ring with his thumb, just as he always has done, a little habit we used to joke was like him counting rosary beads, reassuring him when he was stressed and, he would add with a cheeky wink, 'keeping me on track'.

I looked at his hand, at its familiar curve, seeming just as ready to reach out and grab mine as it was when, giggling with relief at being reunited, we had walked away hand-in-hand from the *I'm a Celebrity* jungle camp. I moved to the side of the bed to hug him – he smelled like Derek, albeit with overtones of antiseptic salve. Everything felt almost normal.

Without thinking, I leaned forward to take his hand in mine, to feel that reassuring warmth which was always accompanied by a little squeeze. But as he felt my touch, he jolted his hand away in panic. His head turned and there was terror in his eyes. Then, realising it was me, he softened and managed an unconvincing smile.

I felt myself go cold. *Did he know who I was?* He'd reacted with terror, followed by a semblance of kindness and childlike hope. He was like a kid thinking someone was his mum and reaching up and finding a stranger. Was he lost in his own world, in his own fears? Had he forgotten who I was? Where he was? I rebuked myself. I knew that I should always ask permission to take his hand. The doctors had told me his body was likely to feel alien to him at times and we knew touch was one of his many sensitivities, along with sound and light. The neurologist wondered if his perceptions were so confused that touch, even gentle touch, might feel like pain. And we were encouraged to help him begin to learn the difference. This was one of the reasons why I wanted to get some kind of relaxing massage and aromatherapy into his life, so he could begin to enjoy being touched by me, the kids and others. Loving touch, as it were, rather than the practical touch of repositioning and physio. It also occurred to me that, when I'd come into the room, I hadn't made my presence known to him, something we were told we should always do.

Because Derek was trapped in bed, immobile, he needed to feel that his room was safe and private. When you have no control over your body, it's important to have control over who comes near, as you have no way of preventing that intrusion into your space. I'd never before had the feeling that he saw my presence as an invasion – he always seemed to light up when I was there. Sometimes he would insist that the carers call me to find out where I was, even when I was on air on *GMB*, and I would have to rush out in ad breaks to reassure him and remind him that I was at work, that I would be coming home soon, and that he really was safe. It was like having an umbilical cord stretching between us.

'Sorry, darling,' I said, 'I should have asked before taking your hand.' It broke my heart that I had to ask permission to cuddle my husband. Was this where we were in our marriage now? I felt it was like some grim nightmarish version of Julia Roberts in *Notting Hill* in that scene when she says, 'I am just a girl standing in front of a boy asking him to love her ...' Except the barrier between us wasn't fame and trappings as it was in the movie – it was the ravages of Covid that were separating us. We were peering at each other, his eyes imploring, trying to hide the shock and fear he had obviously felt, mine imploring too, craving love, trying to overcome the emotional slap of the apparent rejection.

I instantly cursed my selfishness at even having these feelings. I was thinking of myself, of the love I wanted *from* him, the way I wanted *him* to be with *me* and for *me*. I wasn't thinking of him and his utter torture at not being able to express himself the way he wanted to. How could I react like this, like a hurt child?

But I have concluded over the past three years that sickness is selfish. It consumes the person who is afflicted with it as well as infecting those around them with stress and trauma. Those people then need more from other people and lean on them, and they in turn become stressed and the need ripples out. Obviously, it affects the person who is suffering the most. Think about when you have raging toothache, it's all you can think about. It consumes your personality. You might be snappy with people when you wouldn't normally be; it strips away the pleasure you get from things you would usually relish, because it dominates your brain. The purpose of pain is to signal that something is wrong – it's telling you, 'Don't ignore this feeling, this is important!'

Pain can also take over your body processes, I now learn. When you have, say, an infection in one part of your body, your brain focuses on that area to fight it, literally directing energy towards what is most vital for survival. For instance, organs like kidneys sometimes shut down even when they are not directly affected by an illness because the body prioritises the brain and heart first. Very often kidneys are the last organ to recover, too, when the whole body is in crisis. It's the brain ruthlessly focusing on what is most necessary for survival at that point.

Suddenly I realised that all this time I had been staring at Derek but not really looking at him – and that he was gazing back at me, confused.

'Shall I sit with you for a bit?' I said, trying to sound cheery. 'I see you're watching *Life of Brian* – I haven't seen that in years.' I was hoping that looking at something neutral together might relax us both. What I really wanted to say, though, was, 'Let's not look at anything else. Look at *me,* be with me, love me.'

God! Selfish, selfish, selfish.

'Yes please,' said Derek again, smiling that weak, childlike smile. Its sweetness suddenly irked me, disturbed me, but I wasn't sure why. What a horrible, horrible person I must be. Why was I thinking these thoughts? I cringed as I remembered that, as I had left *GMB* that morning and was on my way to the Smooth studio, a lovely woman came up and hugged me. She told me she had been a nurse for 20 years, that I was doing amazingly, that I should keep going. She acknowledged how hard it was to care for others, but also how worthwhile. She had been so kind and I felt as though I was betraying her by even thinking these selfish thoughts. I was certainly betraying Derek.

I looked at him again. He was in his own world, staring at the screen, seemingly comforted by my presence. But *I* couldn't stop *my* internal screams: 'You don't see me! What are we now?'

There had been so many moments when I had just stared at Derek. When he'd been in the coma, I'd watched him on the iPad praying and was talking to him about anything and everything he might hear, hoping he was reassured by my spelling out his future and how wonderful it was going to be. I had told him how much we loved him and missed him, and how proud we were of him, encouraging him to keep fighting for us, and for the kids. I had seen him broken, his body emaciated, staring, unable to even get his eyes to follow me around the room. I would talk to him, waiting for the moment when his eyes would alight on me, when there would be some connection. I had been with him when he'd had to endure agonising tests that made him scream in pain, and when he had pushed himself to continue with therapy, even though we could see that his body was collapsing beneath him, and the pain of even trying was unbearable.

I had seen him nearly slip away from me so many times over the last three years. Only a few months earlier, I'd held his hand as we learned that sepsis could take him once again. When he was crazed with infection, shaking, almost convulsing in a fit. Through all this, I felt we were connected by the incredible strength of love and it could pull us back and pull us through. Even more recently, we'd thought a new infection would take him away from us and again I was with him all night as he fought it. He'd been delirious and hallucinating and seemed not to even know I was there. Each time, I had felt fear, terror and heartbreak. And each time, when I most feared I would lose him, I felt overwhelmed by how much I loved him, and I believed I could sense that he loved me. I felt like his wife, his Kate, and he was my Derek.

But now, for the first time I felt disconnected, estranged, like I'd really lost him, rather than being on the brink of saving him. It wasn't that he was behaving differently; rather, it was my own thoughts and needs that were destroying us. I hated myself, yet I couldn't stop the waves of sadness and fear for our love breaking over me, even after we'd been through so much. Was his love for me real, or did he see me as just another carer? Just a more attentive one. I hated myself for even thinking that could be true – of course that wasn't how he felt. He just couldn't show me anything more right now. The fact that he could trust me to accept him, wasn't that the greatest sign of love? He trusted me with his life. For heaven's sake, he trusted me to make any decision he was unable to – what more could I expect? And yet, in that moment, I wanted more.

I was close to finishing writing this book, and naming it *The Strength of Love,* but was it now my love that was finally failing because I wanted more?

I moved the focus from inside my head, away from these horrible disturbing thoughts, back to Derek. Friends who have had to nurse their loved ones through terminal illness have described how, as their bodies failed, they disappeared inside themselves, apparently not noticing anyone else. For the person who is with them, it is so painful because they can sense their loved one slipping away and, at the very time they want to hold on to them, to feel them the most, it's as if they are turning from them.

I was being selfish by wanting Derek to be, in that moment, the Derek he used to be, the Derek who was focused on me, on us, on our love, on our family, on the life that we have made together. But that wasn't the Derek he could be right now. His body wouldn't let him.

A huge crash, followed by demented-sounding banging on the door, snapped us both out of our trance: Derek from his fixed gaze on the movie, an old friend he was revelling in watching again, chuckling and smiling at its humour; and me from the strange movie running in my head – a terrifying horror film I had never seen before.

'Ah,' I said, realising what the noise was, 'I think that's one of the twits home,' I said. 'Twits' was the affectionate name we gave our kids. He looked at me and said, 'Good.'

It was Bill and of course he ran straight in to see Derek. Bill had never seen *Life of Brian* before, or even heard of Monty Python, so he started asking his dad about the film. I saw that Derek was now distracted by Bill and, trying to sound as breezy as I could, said, 'I'm just going to go and sort out some food before Darcey gets back.'

I went through to the kitchen and started rooting around for ingredients with which to make a chilli, relishing having something practical to do that might take my mind off the dark thoughts of the last half hour. My phone rang: it was my friend Vickie. I almost didn't pick it up as I didn't think I'd be able to hide the state I was in. But I so rarely got a chance to speak to friends. Between caring for Derek, being on air, looking after the kids and everything else, there were so few opportunities to have a catch-up that I couldn't let this one go.

'Wow, this is the triple threat of Kate Garraway experiences!' Vickie said, bursting with excitement. 'I realise I've actually got a missed call from *you*. Normally it's the other way around. Then, I realise you've left a voicemail, which I listen to with trepidation, wondering what dramas have befallen you, only to find that you've had a great week. And now, to top it all, I've called you back and you've *actually* picked up! I can't believe it. I feel like I've won the lottery!'

I felt terrible: she was so happy and caring. I burst

into tears, my heart aching so much that I couldn't even gather myself enough to speak to her.

'Oh my God, what's happened?' She sounded terrified.

'Nothing it's nothing,' I managed to blurt out.

'Clearly, it's not nothing. Take a deep breath, I'm here. Whatever it is, we can get through it.'

She was being so kind, just like everyone else around me. I was surrounded by love: friends, colleagues, bosses ... even strangers I bumped into on the street. I had so much when so many people in my position had so little and were battling on their own. I felt I didn't deserve her support. She just waited and waited while I tried to find the courage to say what I was feeling.

'Whatever it is, don't think about it, just tell me.'

'I'm so ashamed ... I can't.'

'You *can*, you can tell me anything.'

'I'm so lonely!' The words came from nowhere. They hadn't even formed in my head before they were out of my mouth and it was terrifying and shameful to hear myself say them. 'I am so sad and so lonely and I just don't know what to do. I can't save Derek. I think I'm failing the children. I can't make up for the loss of their dad. I'm exhausted but not really from caring. I don't mind that – I feel it's an honour to care for him and I like it because it makes me feel close to him. It's just tonight. I looked at him and felt so alone and I've never felt that before, not since the day I met him, and I don't know what to do with those feelings.'

It felt as though she was silent for a very long time. I actually wondered if she'd hung up.

'Darling, I have never been so happy,' she said, softly and calmly.

'What?'

'I've been waiting for this call for so long. I have been edging you towards this, haven't you realised?'

No, I hadn't.

'Every time I speak to you, you give me a long list of the horrific things that have happened in the last week, and then you say, "but the good thing is ..." and it's always something positive about the kids or about what Derek has been through. And if there's nothing positive to say you tell me that we just have to keep going. All that time I've wanted to scream down the phone, "What about you, darling Kate, what about *you*?" It's all we, your friends, talk about and we know that something's got to give, and we fear it will be you.'

'I know, I know,' I said. 'I've got to keep going, I've got to keep the ship afloat. I feel I'm letting everyone down: the kids, Derek ... I don't know why I'm feeling like this, because I was feeling so happy and positive today. Derek is in a great place at the moment and I can't quite believe that I'm even having these thoughts! Vickie, I'm so sorry.'

I tried to gather myself.

'No, darling, that is the opposite of what I'm trying to say. I don't want you to get yourself together. I don't want you to keep the ship afloat. But I don't want you to break, either, because I'm terrified for your health. You know you can't keep going like this: a few hours' sleep a night, living on adrenaline, trying to advocate for Derek while navigating the care system and all the different parts of the health service. Sometimes I come off the phone to you, Kate, and Nick [her husband] asks me what's going on with you and Derek. I have to tell him that I don't really know because I am so confused by all the different things you talk about, and I feel exhausted just at the thought of it all. I tell him that I'm worried that it's all too much and you're going to get sick.'

I didn't dare tell her at that point that I had in fact been ill and had ended up in hospital – and that even though it seemed to be an isolated incident, the doctors really weren't clear about the long-term diagnosis. Various theories had been put forward: the episode might have been a one-off heart issue that the docs were now keeping an eye on; it might have been stress-related angina, or it could also have my body's response to stress in general. Mind you, by now I was used to medical uncertainty and unsure diagnoses! Whatever it was, I now realised that I hadn't been able to properly recover – not because I wasn't taking my health seriously but because I'd needed to move on to the next drama with Derek and the kids – I didn't feel as though I had a choice.

I hadn't even had a chance to tell Vickie what had happened and that was partly because I didn't want to keep having conversations with my friends about things that would worry them. I wanted to talk to them about positive things and about their lives as well as mine. Vickie was right, though. I really did have to start taking care of myself, not least because other people were relying on me. I couldn't bear the fact that my friends were worrying about me.

'And before you say it, don't think we're talking behind your back in an awful way, it's only because we love you and we are worried for you.'

I started to sob uncontrollably again. 'I feel so awful. I can't believe I am thinking something so selfish and ungrateful.'

As I said these words, I glanced at one of the kitchen surfaces. In among the kids' toys, old papers, bills and typical Kate clutter was a huge, beautiful white orchid. It had been there for a few months, sticking out like a sore thumb, thriving amid the chaos. Elton John had sent it after we'd seen his show. It had been delivered with the most gorgeous handwritten note saying, 'Can't believe that you got to come. David and I were so thrilled. It was so wonderful and the absolute highlight for us after all that we have shared and all that we've seen you go through. You are so inspiring, as is Derek, and we are here whenever you need us.'

Usually, every time I looked at the orchid, my heart leapt as I was reminded how lucky I was to have so many wonderful people sparing the time to send lovely messages. Now, though, I just felt guilty. I didn't deserve this kind of consideration. I didn't deserve anything. I felt like a terrible fraud. I had spent so long thinking about Derek and his survival that I had even forgotten who I was. If I couldn't save Derek, if I couldn't be a loving carer, who the hell was I?

I had never thought this way before and it was frightening; it felt as if my mind wasn't truly my own.

Vickie piped up again.

'Darling, you've got to grieve. Have you not realised yet that you are grieving? You have never given yourself a chance to do that.'

'What do you mean, *grieve*?' I asked. 'Derek is here, alive. That's the whole point. He's right next to me. I spend every waking minute thinking about him and the children. The only break I get is when I'm on air. I think that's why I love my work so much. It's a bit of the old me. There are thousands dealing with real grief every day and they would give their eye teeth to be in my situation.'

'I know, I know,' she said. 'And nobody could love Derek more than I do, except possibly himself,' she teased – and it was a relief to hear some banter.

'True,' I almost laughed.

'It's not that, it's just ...'

But before she could finish, I interrupted, suddenly taking on board the fact that she thought I was grieving that Derek had gone.

'Hang on, you're my chief manifesting mentor. You've

told me that you believe 100 per cent that Derek can recover, that he can come back. Obviously, he'll be changed. We know that – we've all been changed by this – but are you now saying you are giving up on him?'

'No, I'm not. I'm just not sure that he will improve quickly enough for you to get some mental peace. God knows, we are all willing him to get better, and you are doing more than any wife could do. I'm not saying this to make you feel guilty, I just think you should think about maybe taking a step back and taking some time for yourself. It's not that I think he may not improve. It's just that in your drive to save him and never give up, I think you have given up on yourself a bit.'

That hit me like a cannonball.

'God, do you think I've been letting myself go? Do you think I've been bad at my job? Neglecting the kids?'

'You're still missing the point. Stop apologising and stop feeling guilty, it's not helpful. You're the journalist, Kate. Rather than spending every waking moment investigating and managing things for Derek, do some investigating for yourself. And start by looking at grief.'

At that moment Derek pressed his buzzer.

'I've got to go. Derek's buzzing, I need to go and see to him.'

Vickie sighed, 'I know. You've got to go. Promise me you will think about it, though.'

I went to Derek. He smiled and said, 'Where you go? Stay.'

My heart broke again. I couldn't believe I'd been having those awful thoughts. His expression was so warm and loving that they just melted away – it felt like a ghost leaving my body. He was loving me so hard, in the only way he could. How could I ask for more?

I lay next to him on the sofa, beside his bed. He awkwardly stretched out his hand. I put mine in his and we stayed there contentedly until he fell asleep.

Then I went to check on the children. Darcey had helped herself to the chilli and fed Bill too, and they were happily snuggled up, watching TV.

'All okay in here?' I asked.

'Sure … Why wouldn't we be?' Darcey looked puzzled.

'No reason.' They couldn't know that I had just been through a crisis of confidence, this dark night of the soul.

'You okay, Mum?' Bill looked concerned.

'Yes, just tired.' I flopped down in a chair and tried to be normal, looking at the programme they were watching. 'Oh no, she hasn't got you into *Love Island,* too, has she, Bill? I can't have two addicts in the house.'

They visibly relaxed – Mum's normal service had been resumed. While they chatted about the latest twists and turns, I smiled and laughed. We were back.

However, while they were distracted, I subtly picked up my phone and googled 'grief'.

Chapter 10

Am I Grieving?

So, was I grieving? I had never thought of describing what I was feeling – what I and the kids and our wider family and friends were experiencing – as grief. In fact, I had felt I was existing in a state that was the exact opposite of grief. Derek was alive, here, fighting on – we had him with us, when so many millions were dealing with the brutality of bereavement. I could only feel gratitude. And guilt, too, if I was 'having a bad day' or struggling, because this was what I had prayed for – the chance to care for Derek, in whatever state he was in, the chance to fight for him to survive.

Acknowledging any kind of struggle in our lives seemed a terrible betrayal: of this gift, of all the love that had been shown to me and to him, of life itself, in a way. Grief was about loss, wasn't it? We hadn't lost Derek –

he was either next to me or actively in my thoughts, every minute of the day. Even when I was on air, I was always thinking, 'What do I need to do for him about this or that medical crisis? How can I make things better?' In fact, my radio shows on Smooth were frequently punctuated with FaceTime calls from the carer, so that I could share what I was doing with Derek, and he could be reassured by knowing I was with him in some way. However, when I looked up the definition of grief, I began to understand what my friend Vickie meant.

Grief is a complex emotion with many faces. Although most commonly associated with bereavement, it can be triggered by many other types of loss too, like the end of a relationship, or the loss of a job or a home – any event that snatches away the stability of the life you'd had before, and the life you'd planned and hoped would come.

Health changes also involve these kinds of losses, and I could see that Derek must be feeling grief about the state Covid had left him in, and what it had stripped away. Grief for the loss of his ability to do all the things he loved, from his work in psychology and his passionate mental health campaigning, to the simplest everyday things he'd always enjoyed so much, like making the kids their breakfast and playing with them in fun and inventive ways; going for a walk (he used to relish walking into his office in central London in the mornings); chatting and laughing with his friends. Just having the chance to live his life and carry on working to make his dreams real.

Derek is grieving, of course he is – he has lost so much of who he was. He is trapped in a body that speaks to him of his losses night and day, often in the language of pain and discomfort. It would be a nightmare for anyone. And I realised that he must be wondering every minute of the day who *he* was now, what his life was going to be and if the old life, the old Derek, was lost for good. During the times when he was more withdrawn from us, more lost in himself, was he in fact processing some of that grief deep inside? All those who love him could grieve for his loss *for* him, and feel sympathy for what he was going through, but were we also grieving for ourselves?

In her seminal book *On Grief and Grieving*, Elisabeth Kübler-Ross defined the five stages of grief as: denial, anger, bargaining, depression and acceptance. The stages aren't necessarily linear, so you can't expect to move through them in a straightforward way, not like following a road map; you can't be sure how quickly you might end up in a place of calm acceptance, where you can celebrate the love without the pain, but I wasn't sure how to move through them at all. Still, I began to try, starting with denial.

I'm sure many of my friends thought I lived in a constant state of denial, refusing to accept that my life had changed for good. But of course I knew it had changed and I had certainly accepted that there would be no easy return to the life we'd had before. Yet, did that mean I had to give up entirely? It wasn't, after all, as if Derek had actually died. We weren't bereaved. And wasn't my resistance to the continual warnings that he might die part of what had kept us all going, part of what sustained him and kept him striving? It certainly seemed so.

In any case, the constant risk of death and the continual fluctuation in Derek's condition made it hard to know quite what it was I was supposed to be accepting. How could I be clear when everything was so clouded by uncertainty? We lived every moment – and still do, even now – with the risk that he could die. Maybe not to the degree that we experienced in those first few months, when we were repeatedly warned that he might not make it through the next few minutes, the next hour or the next day, but all the questions about the damage Covid had done to him meant he was being rushed back into hospital again and again. It had happened so many times, even in recent weeks, with infections or potentially life-threatening developments, that we could *still* never be sure he wasn't going to die.

I had to wonder whether we were experiencing the 'anticipatory grief' that people sometimes go through when somebody close to them is dying. Often, this is a way for the mind to prepare for actual loss and, although it can't spare you the grief and pain that comes when the worst finally happens, it can be a sort of dress rehearsal for your feelings, making what is to come feel a little less intimidating. Anticipatory grief can be helpful if you're trying to rein in your feelings so that you can guide others, especially children, through what is happening. But it's grim, too, because it's as if you're pre-empting the loved one's death, almost hurrying it along, insensitively, even though that's the last thing you would ever want to do.

I had to stay focused on life, not only on the day-to-day details of caring for Derek but also because there was still so much to believe in and hope for. Denying the risk of death, pushing it out of our minds, and fighting for life has been what's kept us going.

There were ripples of grief, though, and these had spread. Grief had definitely affected Derek's parents, who had been prevented from visiting him early on by Covid restrictions, which they had dutifully and honourably stuck by, to the letter. Knowing more than anyone the risk that Covid posed, they didn't want anyone else to go through what they were, and so they unselfishly put others first. Later, they were prevented from visiting him by their own declining health, which Derek's state, I'm sure, exacerbated. The agony of witnessing what their son was going through, and the fear that he might be taken from them at any moment, has had a devastating effect. And every time we tried to make a plan to take him to his hometown of Chorley in

Lancashire – something Derek desperately wanted to do – we hit an obstacle when either Derek's health, or theirs, took a turn for the worse.

I resolved to keep trying, though, because I knew that it would mean everything for Derek, and for them too, just to be in the same room. It would be painful for both and particularly difficult for his parents, because the reality of Derek's condition would come as a sudden slap, rather than the small daily jabs the kids and I were experiencing. But I was certain it would help all of us, especially them, if we could make it to Chorley because they were missing out on getting to know the 'new Derek'. Their love for him couldn't have been greater, but I feared that absence and distance were making their loss much harder. And my heart ached for their plight.

In my research, I learned that what the kids and I were going through could fall under the umbrella of 'ambiguous loss', a term coined by the researcher Dr Pauline Boss to describe a situation that isn't clear-cut. People experience ambiguous loss when a loved one is missing, but no body is found; or when they 'lose' someone to mental health problems, brain injury, a relationship breakup, addiction issues, dementia or any number of other reasons that might mean their loved one is physically present but emotionally absent. It's the loss you feel when they're no longer 'themselves', no longer behaving in the way that made you love them in the first place, no longer existing in the relationship you had with them before. People also experience ambiguous loss when close friends and family members emigrate to a distant country. 'They may as well be dead,' they think to themselves, in the stage of grief they go through before they (hopefully) set up a weekly Zoom link and start saving to go and visit them. This type of grief can be hugely challenging in a different way from the finite, brutal nature of bereavement.

When Derek first came out of the coma but was trapped in a state of minimal consciousness, he was unable to speak and the only way we knew he was aware of anything outside himself was by watching his eyes 'track' around the room, following us. No one could tell us if this would ever change – if he could ever improve. At the time, I spoke to our good friend, the writer Decca Aitkenhead, who has known Derek since they were both in their twenties. Some years ago, Decca went through the horrific loss of her husband when he drowned while trying to save their son. Her life seems almost unbearable in the light of such grief, but when she rang me to offer sympathy and support, she said, 'I think what you are going through may be worse than what I went through.'

'Christ, how can you say that?' I said. 'You were left with the horror of your husband gone and your two beautiful boys never having the chance to see their daddy again. We have hope; we have Derek here with us, alive.'

'I knew you would say that,' she replied, 'and I'm

not belittling the pain we went through and go through every day, but at least I knew what I was dealing with. There was a ground zero – devastatingly, horrifically, soul-engulfingly painful as it was – and yes, I still feel the pain of that moment every day; but at least I knew what I was up against and we could begin, in time, to start accepting and healing. You are facing "mini deaths" every day and, as far as you know, this could go on forever.'

This was my friend being wonderfully caring and unselfish, offering me sympathy and compassion, reaching out a loving arm to say, 'I know you think I have suffered, but your suffering is valid too.' And it was so good and kind of her. But now I am beginning to understand what she was trying to tell me.

Every day, there are significant moments when Derek is 'present' and in these moments there is so much hope for change. So, one minute I'm cresting a wave of optimism – after he has said something so utterly Derek it makes me think that his old self is just out of reach, hidden under the layers of pain, infection and disability, and if we could just 'unwrap him', by doing one more thing, then more of him would emerge. But the next minute, when he follows that with a blank stare into the middle distance, lost to us once more, I'm plunging back down into the depths and all hope comes crashing after me. The vicious sting of these emotional 'mini deaths' never seems to ease for me – or for Darcey and Billy, which is even more heartbreaking, because it's always so much harder to see your kids go through something than to suffer it yourself.

We had got used to Derek being able to respond with a 'yes' or 'no' at the time, when fatigue hadn't completely overwhelmed him, and we were grateful for it, but whenever he attempted to start a conversation – now *that* was elation! One time I wheeled him into the kitchen and Billy was bouncing a large blue basketball on the kitchen floor.

He looked at us guiltily, knowing he shouldn't really be doing it there. 'Sorry. I, I ...'

Before he could continue, Derek interrupted him. 'Inside, Billy?'

'Yes, Dad!' Billy leapt on his response. 'Sorry, I know I shouldn't be.' He turned to put it away.

'Is it new?' Derek continued. Billy swung back round, beaming.

'*Yes!!!* Yes, it is, Dad. I bought it with my birthday money ... Do you like it?'

Derek looked very serious and swallowed hard again and again, as if he was pumping a bellows, cranking up his throat, trying to make his voice box work and draw his thoughts from deep inside his brain.

'Good, it's good,' he said, looking deflated that those were the only words he could get out. I could tell he wanted to say so much more, but he also managed a weak but warm smile.

Billy didn't seem to notice how few words had come

after such a long wait. Maybe his love filled in the blanks. He immediately started chatting away excitedly, telling Derek about why this particular basketball was so great, bouncing it again and again on the floor and throwing it at a cardboard hoop we'd made and attached to the back door.

'You see, Dad, it's so satisfying! It's got just the right amount of bounce and when it goes into the basket, it's such a sweet feeling.'

'Yes,' said Derek, beaming again.

Then Billy, maybe trying his luck as things seemed to be going so well, or maybe just forgetting Derek's limitations, suddenly suggested, 'Hey, Dad, can I throw it to you? Can you catch it?'

I wanted to shout 'No!!!', panicking at the thought of this heavy ball and how Derek was even going to begin to catch it. But I bit my tongue, not wanting to intrude on the father–son moment, and just hovered there to prevent any injury.

I needn't have worried. Bless him, Billy walked over to his dad in his wheelchair and virtually dropped the ball into Derek's lap with just enough movement and a verbal 'hup' to make him feel like he was catching it. Derek beamed. Then we could hardly believe it as, slowly using his good right hand, he squished it against the weaker left, and lifted the ball up in an attempt to throw it back to Billy, but he couldn't quite do it and it rolled down and fell onto the floor.

'Well done, Dad!' said Billy, with the sort of jubilation that he normally reserved for a winning goal in the FA Cup.

Billy went to pick it up and go again, but that was it – the precious connection had broken. Derek suddenly seemed to disappear, vaporise somehow, his expression glazed, his eyes staring vacantly. Billy's expression had changed too. Our time with him being present had run out.

'Bed,' Derek said, his eyes, wild and fearful.

'Of course,' I said, knowing he was exhausted and overcome, and desperate to lie flat.

When I came back into the room, Billy was slumped on the sofa. 'That was great, wasn't it?' I ventured hopefully.

'Yes, and I don't even mind that it didn't last; I'm not sad in any way,' he said, instantly revealing his sadness.

'I know it's hard,' I said, 'but Dad was really trying. He just can't do it for long. It takes so much out of him. We have to be grateful for the moments we have though, don't we?'

'I know, Mum, I know – I said I was happy, didn't I?'

It was heartbreaking. He was caught in his own little vortex, struggling with extremes of emotion – grateful for the time he'd had with his dad, crushed that it had ended and guilty for wanting more. I wanted to smother him in love and take the pain away, but I knew I couldn't. These 'mini deaths' could only be lived through, survived.

Of course, Billy – and Darcey, too – were far from alone in their torment. In 2022, the Childhood Bereavement network said more than 46,000 under-18-year-olds suffered the death of a parent, and hundreds of thousands were affected by a parent figure who was seriously ill. The same year, the Children's Society estimated that there are approximately 800,000 young carers in the UK, some as young as five years old. Friends have told me that, if they get through it, helping to care for Derek will give Darcey and Bill a profound insight into the struggles of other young carers; it will offer them a perspective on life that will benefit their understanding of others and be a positive influence on them in ways we cannot yet see. But that's only *if* they get through it, while at the same time having (like thousands of others) their education and social lives skewed by the pandemic, and also going through all the stuff that teenagers go through: the insecurities; the fears; the pressure of exams; explosive new feelings. God, I miss you, Derek … This is what you are good at … managing the kids' emotions and giving them that stability.

I was constantly on the lookout for signs of how they were affected, and I worried that what they were going through might lead to depression, one of the stages of grief. I'm very conscious, though, that we mustn't confuse depression with sadness. Derek and the wonderful Ruby Wax have always made clear to me that depression is a very specific neurological condition, which isn't the same as the deep sadness brought on by loss or bereavement, although it can exacerbate it.

What I have learned is that children of chronically ill parents are more likely to internalise feelings of anxiety and deep sadness – and as we all know, a problem that isn't shared can grow like a festering carbuncle inside you. Suppressed feelings have to find a way to come out, whether it's in skin rashes and lumps, or erratic or dangerous behaviour. Teens have trouble regulating their emotions and can be impulsive or snappy at the drop of a hat, so it can be hard to tell whether their moods are being driven by hormones or the effects of trauma. And of course, it's probably a bit of both.

As Bill and I sat there in silence, I felt incapable of helping him. I knew his mind was racing with the same questions as mine; his emotions consuming him, suffocating him, just as mine were. 'Will Dad ever be like he was before?' he asked, purposely not looking at me, staring at the TV screen to avoid eye contact.

'I don't know,' I said honestly. 'We just have to be grateful for what we have, don't we?'

He snuggled into me, not saying anything. Like me, he was grateful for the moments we'd just had, and acutely aware of what we'd lost.

If grief was what we were feeling, I owed it to him and Darcey – and indeed myself – to tackle it head-on.

Chapter 11

Letting Go

O n reflection, telling Vickie that I was tortured by loneliness seemed quite a strange admission, because one of the characteristics of the last three years is that I have not had a single second to myself. Not that I'm complaining, because the presence of people all around us – doctors, nurses, carers, relatives and friends – has been what's kept our family going. But it has left me precious little space to think, to let go and begin to process what we've all been through. I have either been on air or working in other ways; and when I'm not working I'm with the children, indulging in their company while trying to provide for their needs, or I'm caring for Derek or managing his care. But that's the nature of loneliness, isn't it? Sometimes you can be lonely in a crowd – because you're isolated by the pain you are feeling.

I knew, for everyone's sake, I had to lean into this pain in order to begin to heal; but it felt impossible to find a space to do it, because taking 'time out for myself' would have meant letting others down: not making that vital call or not being at the hospital when I was needed. It would have meant not attending that meeting with the care administrators so that I could keep pushing for them to continue the life-saving support Derek needed. Or not going into work. Or not spending time with the children, who also really needed my support. Or not being with Derek, who clung to me more and more as a reassuring presence.

Then, almost by accident, the opportunity to get some time to myself opened up in the strangest of ways. My great friends Chris Hawkins, BBC 6 Music presenter, and his wife Clare Nasir, my friend from *GMTV* who is now Channel 5's meteorologist, had insisted a year earlier that we put a date in the diary so that Derek, Darcey, Billy and I could have a break with them and their daughter, Sienna, at Chris's dad's disabled-friendly holiday bungalow in Abersoch, Wales. At the time I'd smiled wistfully at the thought, but loved their positivity and saw power in the idea that we were setting a date. It was a fixed point to aim for, a way of manifesting the chance for us all to be together. It was a wonderful idea – even though Derek's constantly variable state of health, and all the risks each day brought, made it seem like an almost impossible fantasy.

Of course, when the date came around, the predictable happened and Derek was back in hospital; another element of Covid damage had unravelled his progress and, on top of that, he had another serious infection that again threatened his life. I left a voicemail message for Chris and Clare, saying, 'I'm so sorry, I'm going to have to let you down again. Derek is back in hospital, he needs an operation, and I don't feel I can leave him to go as far away as Wales. I'm so sorry not to be there and the kids will be crushed too, they were really looking forward to it.'

When they didn't call back, I was worried that I had pushed them too far and tested the limits of our friendship by letting them down at the last minute. But then my mum called and said that she had been talking to Clare and Chris and that they had decided between them that the kids and I really needed to go away. I started to explain that I couldn't, but she interrupted me and said, 'No, you have to. We've arranged it all. I know that you can't go immediately, but the kids can and you can join them after Derek's operation and at least have a couple of days away. Di [Derek's sister] is going to come down to be with him.'

No matter how many objections I raised, she had an answer for all of them and, actually, I couldn't have been more grateful, not least because it meant the kids wouldn't miss out on getting away, because of course we'd not been anywhere since Derek first got sick.

Clare came down to collect Darcey and Billy and they went off happily with their packed lunches, chatting away and excited about the trip, giving me a chance to focus on Derek for the rest of the day. The next morning Di arrived. Derek's infection was receding and he was recuperating on a general ward so I felt safer to go, but he still needed someone to visit and reassure him. I handed her all the instructions about what she needed to keep an eye on and what to take to the hospital for him. 'Stop panicking! We will be fine and if I forget something, I will call you. It's Wales, not Mars!'

At Euston station, I nervously boarded the train to Bangor. It was only as we pulled out that I realised this was the first time I had been physically on my own since Derek got sick. I've always thought there was something wonderfully romantic about trains. It's mesmerising to sit back and watch the countryside roll out before your eyes, especially on a long journey – even more so when a busy, dirty metropolis like London gives way to vast landscapes and skies.

I texted Di to check that things were going well and she assured me that all was fine. Derek was resting and she had even managed to help him have a sip of hot chocolate. I thought of his vulnerable face, of him cautiously attempting the simplest of tasks, and tears welled up in my eyes. The image in my mind seemed a world away from the man I had first met, from the Derek I had married.

Letting Go

It's very hard to pinpoint what you love most about someone or to determine what extraordinary change or event might break your feeling of attachment. People say 'I just knew' about the moment they fell in love – it's a connection, a click or a dopamine fizz that can only be explained up to a point by brain doctors or relationship experts. Twenty years down the line, when the first giddy hook-up has solidified into contented attachment, how do a happy couple describe what they have? Is it bigger, deeper, thinner, less imbued with emotion than it used to be? Is it just habit, taking comfort in the familiar, the trappings of life that we surround ourselves with, a kind of compatibility – that one person's skills or needs luckily fit with yours? Is it in any way definable? And, if so, what is that definition?

I knew that what I was about to do would be like torturing myself but I sensed this was the moment that I needed to push myself to the limit. I called Derek's old mobile number and heard his 'old voice' on the answerphone – so powerful, so in control, the soft Lancashire accent so familiar and now so distant from the whispered words we heard from Derek every day. Already I was floored, but knew I had to push on and go deeper, so I searched his last texts to me and his emails going further back than the final heartbreaking ones he'd sent me from the hospital, before he was put into the coma.

These were emails from 2019 and early 2020. Some

were very practical – the sort of thing you might pin on the fridge: 'Pick up X' or 'I can't make that. Can you?' Then there were lengthier ones about the children – about Darcey's GCSE options and Bill's struggles with maths; and there were others about me – the way things were going with my projects I was beavering away at.

'What you've written, darling, is really good. I am having a good day too but will tell you about that later over your famous Thai fish cakes for tea tonight – hint hint?!' he'd written.

At the time, I had seen these messages in an almost businesslike way. As I rushed around, busy with work and the kids, I would respond, 'That's fine' or 'No no, sorry, no can do.'

Three years on, reading these day-to-day conversations brought me to tears. I felt full of regret that I hadn't treasured this connection, this easy communication, more. Everything was there, in a handful of emails representing the heart and purpose of my life. If someone had asked me to explain what it was that Derek and I had together – how we loved and why our relationship worked – I could have sent them these few notes of love and support, of care for the kids and affection for each other and our family, and that's all they would have needed to see. An easy exchange, where we didn't need to explain ourselves. To other eyes perhaps his words would have looked blunt, but not to mine because I 'just knew'.

How much of the old Derek remained? Just asking that sent me diving into the question of who Derek was before he became ill, and whether it was possible to define him precisely in that way – and whether you can ever truly define anyone? Clearly, identity is fluid: we grow and develop over time; our sense of self changes; we lean in and out of different characters and situations. And yet people talk about core identity, the essence of us, the part that is unique and individual – so perhaps I was really asking, 'What is the core of Derek Draper?'

When we first met, Derek came in a package with colourful stories attached, including all the dramatic, laudable and disastrous things he'd done in his career in politics, before I knew him. He was this loud, entertaining person, to the extent that his friends would tell tales of his exploits in a way that made him seem almost like a mythical figure! I'm sure not all of them were true but the stories people told about Derek always ended with the words, 'He's brilliant, though, isn't he?'

The first time I saw him, though, I wasn't drawn to *that* Derek Draper, or at least not solely. There was another side to Derek that I saw – a thoughtfulness, maybe even a sadness. He had been through so much and, yes, he definitely still had purpose and wit and quick repartee, but also a kind of searching, which I found intriguing, as it seemed so different from his reputation. Maybe he was still haunted by his breakdown and the period of depression that had led him to finish with politics and start a new life, the kind of life he really wanted. He'd only been back in the UK for a few weeks when we met, having retrained as a psychologist and psychotherapist at the Wright Institute in Berkeley, California. So he was busy finding a place to set himself up in practice, just as we got together.

As well as being clever, he was an utter buffoon, a bit like a sharp-witted court jester. But when he was in business mode, he was just brilliant. So he came with a reputation as a genius; maybe a flawed genius, but ultimately someone whose brain was his friend. Whenever anyone described him from his past in politics before I knew him, whether they loved or hated him – and there were plenty of both! – they always said, 'He's so furiously clever' or 'He has a big brain.' His intelligence seemed to define him.

But if there was a question about whether his brain was irretrievably damaged, that also raised the question, 'Was Derek still Derek Draper, if he was no longer "clever"?' And what did that mean for our relationship?

Whenever we discussed things, he always seemed to interpret the world in a unique way that was often very different from mine. I loved that; it was exciting, exhilarating – and sometimes infuriating! I got things that he didn't, and he got things that I didn't. It felt as if, together, we were more than the sum of our parts. We made each other think better, further and more deeply about life.

We were always united in our love of family and our love of the children – that was at our core and I knew that part of us remained. You only had to see the flicker of light in his gaze when he looked at the children to realise that. Of course, he couldn't engage with them in the way he used to; he couldn't be the father he used to be and the three of them lived with the pain of that. Both sides trying, both sides hurting.

In the autumn after we met, in 2004, I was the one that got sick. I suffered repeated kidney infections which kept landing me in hospital, and I had a lump on my kidney, which turned out to be a cyst, but which the doctors had feared could be a cancerous tumour. I was in hospital for a month as they tried to deal with the infection, and ultimately I had the cyst removed and tested and fortunately it was benign. This time together fast-forwarded us from casual dating to a deeper, more serious relationship.

We had planned to get married in May 2006 but we brought it forward to September 2005, exactly a year to the day we met, because I found out I was having a baby. Or, as we would later put it, 'Darcey Draper had decided she wanted to arrive and she wasn't prepared to wait!' We were delighted, obviously.

We had a conversation about whether we should wait to be married until after she'd arrived, which would have been March 2006, and Derek said, 'No, I think we should just go for it, because after she's here, it will be different. This way, we can have one day in September that's for the two of us before we go into family life.'

So we went for it: we were married and very quickly went from being a couple to being a family unit.

In our marriage, it was very much yin and yang. When you think you're going to lose someone, there's often a tendency to look at everything through rose-tinted spectacles, but I was very aware that our relationship wasn't perfect. We were just lucky that our flaws seemed to fit together in a way that made us both better; we could tolerate each other, and somehow make up for what the other one lacked. So, despite its imperfections, it was perfect for us. We fitted around each other really well. Derek was super-organised. He was on top of finances and bill paying; he would plan and book our holidays. It wasn't that he took over; he would always say, 'What do you think about this?'

I'd say, 'Great!' because I really didn't mind; whatever we were doing, I always knew that he would have thought through whether it worked for the kids, and I would just be happy with us being together. He would take charge of creating time for us – date nights were such bliss! It felt like a real treat to see a film with subtitles in a fancy cinema or drink cocktails at the St Pancras Hotel Bar, chatting animatedly all the way home.

It was Derek who really drove our family life. I would do the cooking and the cleaning and make sure we had food in the fridge – plus, of course, I was doing 50 per cent of the earning. Having a family involves quite a few circus skills: balancing, juggling, tightrope walking but, between us, we somehow managed to make it work. The circus tent occasionally flapped in the wind, but it never came down.

As I've said, Derek was very funny and good with words – he loved puns and wordplay. Because of his breakdown, and because of the therapy he'd been through, he was also very good at accessing emotion and communicating it, which is a fantastic quality to have in a partner. And when it was *me* who was stressed, he was very good at letting me know that I should ask for help.

On the other hand, whenever Derek was stressed or worried about something, he had a pattern of behaviour: take it out on me and then get cross about something that didn't seem relevant. When he did this, I'd realise that something more was going on for him and would give him the time and space to process whatever it was. Eventually, he would come back and say, 'It wasn't really about that.'

I'd say, 'I know. What was it about? How can I help?' and we'd discuss it.

Early in our relationship, there was a bit of a turning point when we had our first row. I had turned up really late one evening because I had been held up at work – it had got later and later, and I'd texted Derek to let him know I was running late and I'd meet him at his house.

Eventually – and it really was quite a long time later – I arrived.

'Okay, there is something you need to know about me,' Derek said. 'I don't mind if you say you're late. I don't mind if you say you can't make it. But leaving me feeling anxious, not knowing whether you're coming or not, will make me mad. You've made me really cross.'

'Oh, I'm sorry!' I said, but 'sorry' wasn't enough.

'No, these expectations are really important to me,' he insisted.

I couldn't see why he was so annoyed. I had a reason for being late, didn't I? I was being completely honest when I said, 'The problem was, I couldn't do anything about it because it was sliding out of my control. And I didn't want to cancel because I knew if I didn't see you tonight, then I wouldn't see you before I had to go away ...'

'That's all fine,' he said. 'But now you've just got to front it up and deal with the anger.'

It was classic Derek: everything was out in the open, cards on the table, no confusion.

I got really upset, thinking that because he was so cross he was going to break up with me, that he didn't want to be part of my crazy life. And it *is* crazy when you're a reporter: you get phone calls at all hours, and you have to rush off here, there and everywhere chasing a story. While I had got used to living like this, I could see how difficult it would be for him.

By now it was really too late to do anything, so I went home.

I wondered what the future held for us – and whether he would forgive me and, in the longer term, whether he'd be able to cope with the self-centredness that came with my career and my having lived on my own for so long. Would he give me a chance to build the loving relationship I really wanted and have the family I craved? I suppose I wanted to know if he could tolerate enough of my flaws and give me the space to be vulnerable, to cede a bit of my independence and expose myself to the risk of falling in love. It wasn't conscious, but I think, back then, I was asking him to fight for me, just as I now believed I was fighting for him, and for our family.

The following day, he put a CD through my door. The CD was Bob Dylan's 'Make You Feel My Love', an epically romantic love song that makes your skin tingle as you listen to it, even when your boyfriend *hasn't* given it to you after a row. There was an accompanying note saying, 'Can we talk?'

We did talk. 'I think your problem, Kate, is that you think everything has to be perfect and if something goes wrong, you won't be accepted,' Derek said. 'I'm not saying things don't go wrong. I'm not saying I won't be angry, but I am saying that I'm not going to go away. So, don't think you have to avoid conflict and make everything perfect. Just because I'm cross, I'm not going to leave you.'

Thinking about all this in the empty train carriage, I said out loud, 'But you sort of *have*, haven't you, Derek? That Derek isn't present right now and I miss him so much!' Thank goodness there was no one to hear this crazy woman talking to herself, cursing and crying!

No sooner than I'd said it, I felt guilty. Disloyal. I knew that Derek was still there and I would never stop trying to help him but I also knew that I had to acknowledge that, right now, he couldn't be there for me in the old way. And I had to somehow find a way to live with that in order to feel some peace and allow him to heal in the way he needed to emotionally, even if that meant him withdrawing. To love him as he is – and not dwell on what he was – would free him to be the person he is now. I knew I needed to work on myself, to be happy for myself, and not constantly let my mood be dictated by whether Derek was having a good day or a bad day. Somehow, I had to untie my own emotional stability from his health. There was no doubt that our bond remained strong, woven with love and care, but it had to allow us to be the people we are now. And I knew this meant I had to do some work on myself.

There had been a shift in our relationship, because I am caring for him – it was no longer equal. At times it almost feels like a mother–child dynamic and I can't help missing and craving our old partnership – the fact that he used to be stronger and do so much for me. And there's the sadness that the old relationship between Derek and the kids isn't there any more.

Who was the new Derek and how much of the old Derek remained? For once I couldn't really look to science for answers to these questions. Even if we'd had up-to-date scans, which we didn't, it could never be as simple as comparing the 'Before' with the 'After'. Human beings are infinitely complex because of the size and intricacy of their brains, and the systems and networks that spark and zap within them. Even the most expert neurologist can't tell you precisely what makes these networks function as they should, or what exactly happens when they go wrong.

As our knowledge of the human genome increases, we're getting closer to an understanding of brain function. In the meantime, have you ever seen a photograph of brain cells? They are unfathomable in their beauty, like the Milky Way, like a phosphorescent sea or a cloud of fireflies at night. And we know so little about them that I can't imagine there will ever be a time when we can look at a patch of brain matter in a scan and say, 'Ah yes, this damaged area will affect his ability to find slapstick funny; he won't cry at footage of baby polar bears anymore.' It just isn't like that.

As I sat alone, gazing at the beautiful views through the train window, the emotions just kept coming with a power that was disturbing but strangely also felt right. Guilt, shame and finally anger, the anger that everybody said I should have been expressing for a long time, the anger that I know Derek would have forced me to express. Real anger, this time, not just frustration at the uncertain nature of Derek's condition and how, because the doctors were having to learn all the time, their ability to help was so limited. This was real fury. My face went bright red. *Why?* I wanted to scream, why did this happen to us? Why did this happen to him? His brain has always been his friend, the thing that has got him out of trouble and kept him going, and now it's his enemy. I was furious with myself for not being able to fix it, even though I knew it had never been in my power to do so. I was crushed, feeling an abject failure, not worthy of the praise people kept giving me for keeping going.

I hated myself too. I didn't like the person this situation had turned me into. It felt as though all I did was battle and fight and push to get help and support for Derek. I never seemed to have time, real time, for anyone or anything, not even for Derek, in truth. I just existed in a frazzle that wasn't helping anybody. I was ashamed of the unbelievable amount of debt we were in. It terrified me. I'd had to accept that Derek's company needed to close because there was no way he could return to it any time soon, if ever; I was struggling to pay off the debts from that but was determined to do so. I was also trying to pay for all that Derek needed to keep going. There never seemed to be enough time to get on top of everything or enough money to go around, and I feared for our family's future. I was angry with myself and I also felt guilty because I knew I had so much, and others were struggling even more.

The coaches rattled along, and if you've ever travelled that route to Bangor you'll know how beautiful it is, and in the final stages of the journey, you are right up against the coastline. The sight of the sun on the water, sparkling against the heavy dark clouds, purple with the promise of some classic Welsh rain, was so beautiful it took my breath away and brought me out of my self-indulgent explosion of emotion, back into the real world.

I checked my phone. Di had texted to say that all was still good. Phew. I realised that the guard had been walking up and down the carriages and now he caught my eye.

'Are you okay?' he asked. 'I've been a little bit worried about you.'

Gathering myself, I apologised. 'I'm so sorry,' I said, trying to sound jovial. 'I think there must've been a lot of stuff in me that needed to come out. I'm just sorry that I had to be on your train! I'm glad the carriage is empty!'

He laughed and said, 'Don't worry about it. We've all been there, sometimes you just have to let it all go.'

He was so kind and wise. He added, 'You're never alone in feeling sad. We all feel that way at times and it's always better out than in!'

I felt enveloped in these loving words from a stranger and gathered myself to meet up with the kids.

When I got to the house, it was deserted. There was a note on the door saying, 'We are at the beach and we've hired a boat. You'll have to swim out to us and come and join us and *leave your phone behind!!!!*'

I followed their directions down to the beach and looked out for a large yellow windbreaker that they said marked their camp. I got into my swimsuit and peered into the distance. About 300 yards from the shore, I spotted the hire boat they'd described. I waded into the water and started swimming. Anyone who saw me on *I'm a Celebrity* will know that speedy swimming is not my strong point! But there was something wonderful about the icy cold water, sweeping around me, making my skin tingle. I remembered the power of connecting with your physical self through your senses because it was something I thought a lot about with Derek, trying to stimulate him, to draw him out of himself and help him manage his emotions. I realised, though, that this moment was the first time I'd thought about it for myself – I was getting in touch with myself again in the most tangible way. I revelled in the water slipping through my fingers, and the tingle in my toes and loved the fact that, because nobody knew I was here, I didn't have to rush.

I had brought my snorkel. I love snorkelling, and as I made my way out to the others, I plunged my head under, submerging myself in a whole new world. Of course, this was no Red Sea dive so there were no shoals of sparkly tropical fish to entrance me, but it's amazing

Letting Go

how even seaweed that looks grotty when it's just lying on the rocks looks magical under the water. It was upright in columns, floating, flowing, and it felt like I was swimming through an underwater cathedral.

I was lost in the extraordinary ordinary, marvelling at it, and for once I didn't immediately think 'Oh, Derek would love this' as I usually did about every new and beautiful experience. There I was, submerged and beginning to find a way of revelling in beauty, just for myself. Thinking about it now, that seems selfish, but I've also come to realise since that it's a gift available to everyone. I guess for too long my mood had depended on how Derek was, and what I could do to make him feel better. I realised now that, ultimately, I can't control that, although I'm determined to try. But the thing I *could* control was my own state of mind and I resolved to do more of the things that gave me happiness, so that I could keep my positivity and energy up, which would enable me to keep ploughing on.

When times are tough and you can't get rid of the 'bad stuff', sometimes the only way to get through is to do more of the good stuff, as my fantastic friend Carla Romano (former *GMTV* L. A. Correspondent) always says. It's like having a glass of water when you are thirsty and noticing that there are loads of bits floating in it. You have two choices: either spend the next few hours trying to pick out every speck of dirt as you get thirstier and thirstier and more and more frustrated; or fill it with so

283

much clean fresh water that it starts to overflow, pushing out the dirt so you don't even see it any more.

As I came closer to the boat, I could hear screams of joy. Darcey, Billy and Sienna were leaping off the side and plunging into the water, then swimming back and doing it all over again. I instantly thought of the wonderful holidays we'd had with Derek and felt a surge of sadness that he couldn't be here because I knew how much he would want to be, more than anything in the world. Derek would never just wander down the steps to get into the water. He always ran and jumped into the pool, trying to make the biggest splash possible.

I watched Darcey and Billy, completely free, leaping and laughing in the water, and I hesitated to call them. I didn't want to break their blissful enjoyment. I didn't want to suddenly appear, like a gloomy shadow on the horizon, a reminder of the sadness, the worry back home. It's like when people ask me 'How are you?' I never really want to answer fully and honestly, because who wants to be the sad one all the time, bringing everyone down, like the weeping widow at the wedding?

As I watched them, treading water, I almost decided to swim back but then they spotted me.

'Mum!!!' screamed Darcey in delight. 'Get on board!' Billy was distracted, shouting at Chris, 'Film me, film me!'

I swam closer, and then Billy saw me. 'Look, Mum, I am "doing a dad" – I can't wait to show him the video!'

And with that, he ran and cannonballed into the sea.

At that one moment, I realised his dad *was* with him, the dad before and the dad now. He had fused them, and both were bringing him joy. Maybe this had partly happened because I hadn't been there to overprotect, or fuss or project my worries; or maybe it was happening anyway, and I had just needed this space to see it. I finally realised I didn't have to fix everything. I just had to keep loving and keep going. Somewhere on that long train journey, and during this life-affirming swim, I had let go and found perspective.

Chapter 12

Work in Progress

O f course I couldn't rely on Derek to lift me up in the way he once had, even though that's what I was craving. It was all he could do to sustain himself.

I've always believed that someone can only ever bring to a relationship what they arrive with. For example, if someone has commitment issues and hasn't really dealt with them, there's nothing you can do to suddenly make them feel ready to commit. If they aren't comfortable in expressing their emotions – or even in touch with their feelings – they are not going to be able to share their emotions and feelings with you. In the past, I'd not really taken this on board and would see a partner's failure to commit, to express emotions (or do whatever it was that was frustrating me at the time) as something I needed to try to improve by making myself more appealing, more desirable in their eyes, as though their challenges were my fault. I then came to understand that while we do indeed all bring our own flaws, fears and issues to relationships, the dream is that two people can work through them together. It doesn't always play out this way, of course, because everyone is on their own timeline and I realise now that the timing hadn't been right in many of my previous relationships.

As I pondered this, I began to understand that this was where Derek and I were right now – I knew he loved me but I also knew it wasn't the right time to expect our relationship to be what we'd always hoped it was. Nobody was to blame and I had to accept I couldn't just fix it. I had to find a way of taking control of my own happiness alongside caring for Derek, and allowing him the space to be who he was right now.

I was starting to realise that it wasn't fair on anyone to look at our current situation through the lens of the past. To keep hoping that we could reclaim parts of what we'd once had, even if it wasn't possible long term, wasn't going to make anyone happy in the here and now. I had to find a way of loving what we had now. It could no longer be about trying to get the 'old Derek' back; it was about connecting with Derek in the present and finding a way to define the relationship we have today.

I knew he loved me – it was just that, at this moment, he couldn't love me in the way I wanted. Hopefully we would one day get to a point where he could, but I knew I couldn't continue in this vacuum. I needed to take some positive action – not just for me, but also for Derek and the kids.

The first thing I did was to write a list of all the things I wanted to be different and then crossed out what I knew was totally out of my control. Looking at what was left, I asked myself what could I realistically affect? Could I do anything to speed up Derek's painfully slow recovery? I could certainly support it but any real change had to come from medical progress and from within himself. Could I really take away Darcey and Billy's pain? I could support and love them but as for filling the gap in their lives left by Derek's state, the painful truth was … not really.

The only power I truly had was over myself. For example, I could try to get on top of our finances, which had been left in chaos by the collapse of Derek's company (I'd had to finally admit that there was nothing I could do to save it). I couldn't stop my family and friends worrying about me but I could try to take the pressure off them by focusing more on my own physical health and emotional equilibrium.

I decided that giving myself mental space to process all this wasn't something that should be restricted solely to snatched moments like that train journey to Wales. Somehow, I needed to weave the space into my everyday existence, even though my life was already suffocatingly crammed with just getting by. So I started slowly to put in place some rituals and techniques to help me achieve a mindset that would, ultimately, help us move forward. These practices have enabled me to approach my life as it is now in a more positive way; and I hope some of you will find that you can take something positive from these techniques too.

I spoke to a friend of mine, Dr Gouri Maher, who practises Reiki and has been supporting Derek throughout his illness. Derek had always been a huge fan of Reiki and that had encouraged me to look into it more. One of her techniques, which I have found really powerful, helps when you are feeling overwhelmed: you simply look up at the sky and take in its expanse. I've found that this soothes my soul and, what's more, you can do it anywhere with a window: at home, on the bus – or, in my case, on the back of a taxi bike! The trick is just to look up and marvel at the infinite space above you.

Dr Gouri then taught me to think of this sense of infinity as contained inside my own mind. Did you know that no one has ever been able to calculate how many brain cells we actually have? There are so many of them, we just don't have the capacity to measure it. I am learning to perceive that this means we are all part of infinite time and space, as a way of helping me put things into perspective. In those moments when our brains might be full of anxious thoughts, our bodies might be confined or afflicted, we can take deep breaths in and out and let ourselves know that we do have the time and space to just 'be'.

Tapping into this sense of possibility has helped me recalibrate my approach to sleep, too. Of course it's fairly routine for me to be up in the early hours of the morning for *GMB* and now with my extra caring responsibilities, I frequently don't get to sleep early enough – as I get into bed, I look at the clock and have a little panic that I have to be up in just a few hours. I now choose to reframe this and reassure myself that those few hours are exactly the amount of time I need to recuperate – all I need to do is relax, close my eyes and allow my body to do the rest. Although I might not be getting as much sleep as I would like, by calming any anxiety about how finite that time is, I free my mind and body to heal and restore in the space that I do have.

I also wanted to give myself space to try to restore the free sense of joy I used to have with friends and colleagues. Naturally, when they haven't seen me for a bit, they caringly want to ask how things are going with Derek and, because I know them so well, my first instinct is to try and bring them up to speed. Given the constantly fluctuating and unpredictable nature of Derek's health, it often feels as though I'm delivering a barrage of negative news. As I see the look of horror spread across the other person's face, it strikes me that my updates are basically ruining their day and they are struggling to know how to respond. Consequently, I feel bad and before I know it, the whole interaction starts to feel tragic. So I quickly add something upbeat, like, 'But there are lots of positive things that have happened too!' Or 'There are so many who passed away – so we know how lucky we are to still have him with us.'

It was Ben Shephard who spotted that I always sought to find a positive in our situation when I was telling people about it. He remarked that talking about it in this way must in itself be helpful. In focusing on the positive – even for the sake of saving a friendship! – I was almost unconsciously affirming that positivity to myself.

This was all true, but I needed to do more – I wanted to supercharge that positivity. How could I make this happen? I did two things. Firstly, I challenged myself with a really hard – but ultimately life-changing – practice. I decided I wouldn't let *any* negative thought enter my mind for a whole week. Let me give you an example. Something happens which means that Derek is sick and has to go back into hospital. Whereas previously my brain would have processed this information and then fast-forwarded to the possible outcomes (what's next, is Derek going to die?), I now choose to simply do what the situation demands of me on a practical level, instead of catastrophising about things that haven't happened yet and over which I have no control. I have been trying to concentrate on what is within my gift to achieve in the present moment: 'We're going to hospital. Right, I will organise the mobility vehicle.'

I try to foster stoicism – I can't control the outer world but I can change how I respond to what is being thrown at me. For a whole week, whenever any negative thought entered my head, I consciously decided that I wasn't going to think about it. When I left the house every morning, I learned to let go of the worry that someone else might not do exactly what I thought they should be doing for Derek. Or if I was stuck in traffic on the way to *GMB* or Smooth, I tried not to think about the consequences of that – of being late for work or letting people down. I couldn't change what was happening and, rather than worrying about it, I would use the time to do something else, even if it was just staring up at the sky or out of the car window. If I could see there was a huge queue for the canteen at the Smooth studio, instead of panicking that I wouldn't get my cup of tea and be on time for my show, I paused and said to myself, 'Don't think that thought. Use the time in the queue to do something useful like using your phone to look for stories that you could use in the show.'

When you actively do this for a while, firstly you realise how often negative thoughts creep in; you then realise that *not* thinking about the negative doesn't affect the outcome. For so long, I'd been thinking of myself as a goalkeeper and that if I turned away for just a moment, the ball would plunge into the back of the net. When I stopped letting the negative thoughts in my head, it helped me to let go a little and I could focus on what Derek and the kids really needed.

While it's not realistic to be positive all the time,

whenever your brain is clouded by a negative thought or worry, if you can commit to the practice for, say, a week then it does start to shift your mindset and reduce the exhausting negative chatter going on in your head. Sometimes, of course, you have to face up to bad things and tackle difficult or unpleasant emotions and situations but I have found that if I start to become mired in the bad stuff, I can turn that around by forcing myself to end every troubling thought in my head with, 'But magically...' and find a positive way to bookend that feeling. It's a neat little tool.

I've been making the kids do this too, which they find funny – and they've begun to turn it to their advantage in ways I didn't intend. For instance, Darcey phoned me to say, 'Mum, I'm going to be really late home and I'm afraid I've used that money I was supposed to spend on schoolbooks getting my nails done. *But magically*, my nails do look amazing!'

'Okay, Darcey,' I replied. 'You do have to take some responsibility, you can't use this as an excuse. When you get home we'll talk about how we find that money that you were supposed to have spent on your schoolbooks!'

I'm also trying to rewire my brain to trust itself so that I feel like less of a failure. You can do this by setting yourself a realistic challenge and then committing to completing it. One trick that helps with this rewiring is never to hit the snooze button. Let me explain: if you press the snooze button when your alarm goes off, it's like admitting that you never intended to get up at the time you set your alarm for – and that the reason for you getting up now isn't as important as you thought it was the night before. So every time you do that, your brain learns that your intentions aren't real and unconsciously logs that it's not necessary for you to do what you say you are going to do – you are unwittingly wiring your brain to accept that you have no power to succeed. And definitely don't set the alarm if you don't actually want to get up because you're setting yourself up for failure!

I realised that I had been doing this and that it wasn't serving me well. On mornings when I didn't need to get up at 2am to do *GMB*, I was setting my alarm for 5am, so that I could get up and finish a task I hadn't completed the night before, thinking I would feel better about doing it the next morning. The truth was, though, that I wanted to put it off and would then beat myself up for not achieving it. It's much better to accept that you need the rest and not set an early alarm in the first place.

I have been trying to reprogramme myself on the days when I do get up early even when work doesn't require me to. As well as actually tackling the task I might be dreading, I also build in time to indulge in activities that are not on my urgent list; I give myself the gift of time to do something which helps only me. It might be only ten minutes of something physical such as stretching, ten minutes of something that delights me (usually pottering in the garden with a mug of tea), ten minutes of reading something stimulating that *isn't* work!, ten minutes of organising myself – and of course ten minutes of the task I most dread as that will ease the guilt I feel around not doing it.

This was a way of actively creating a space where I could find my own peace and happiness, alongside supporting Derek. I realised that Derek also needed distance from me to develop his sense of self in his new state. Our connection was not in question – he was always reassured by my presence – but he needed to be stimulated by other things too. I understood that I had to stop trying to protect Derek so much on an emotional level. The carer still FaceTimes while I'm at work to show me Derek doing his exercises. I love that because I know how much it means to Derek but when it comes to an end, I now actively think, 'This is over now. He's now sleeping safely with the carer. So I'm going to put all my focus on what I'm doing at Smooth, enjoy the music and think about my communication with the listener and really enjoy that experience.'

Finding ways of helping each of us to develop was something I knew I needed to work on. I had to consciously reassure myself that, by looking for new ways forward, I wasn't abandoning the past – rather, I was helping us to forge new identities alongside each other. During my ten-minute sessions in the morning, I would listen to music that I would never have dreamed of listening to before so that I could create a new experience for myself. Previously, Derek and I would have chosen to watch a TV programme that we both liked but now there are certain kinds of shows that he can't watch. Probably because he is still processing his own trauma, he isn't able to watch anything with violence in it (not that he particularly revelled in violent dramas before, but he did love a good Scandi noir detective series). While still inhabiting a shared space, which is what we both wanted, I encouraged us both to explore our tastes now.

When the kids and I returned from that trip to Bangor, I noticed that the children had, in their own ways, started to relate to Derek differently. They were growing up, so it wasn't surprising that the dynamics were shifting – Darcey was 13 years old when Derek first got sick and she was now a young woman of 17. I noticed that she would step in quite naturally to support him in a way that had changed from the early days of his return home. For instance, she delighted in preparing and cutting up his food, and helping him to safely eat it. If I left the room or watched from afar, they would start communicating with each other in a way that was very different from before but no less tender. Gradually, they were finding a new way to be dad and daughter. Bill's relationship with Derek started to redefine itself too, as Bill began to joke and tease him in a way that felt more natural, like he was no longer scared to be a normal teenager for fear of upsetting him. While it's been excruciatingly painful for them to experience everything I've written about in these pages, I could see that they were coming to a place of acceptance and there was a sense of moving forward.

Seeing this made me understand that I needed to push Derek to see his friends. I knew he wanted to but that he was fearful of their reaction. So much had changed and it wasn't going to be easy for either side – and a part of me worried that perhaps after a visit or two they might slip away, unable to cope. I couldn't bear the thought of that happening in case Derek was hurt so it had been easier to allow arrangements to be kicked into the long grass when Derek said he was too tired to see anyone, reassuring myself that it would happen 'one day'.

His friends had always been there for him, though. One day at home, I sat with Derek and we listened to some of the messages that friends had sent for us to play to him while he'd been in his coma. There was a message from Gordon Brown reminding him of the Labour slogan, 'Things can get only better' and from Peter Mandelson and Tony Blair, who talked about the powerful moments they'd shared. It wasn't just his old Labour friends who got in touch, though, there were messages from all sides of politics: Boris Johnson and other members of the Conservative Party, as well some Liberal Democrats all sent him their best wishes.

Other moving messages came from those he'd

encountered through his psychotherapy work. One former newspaper editor rang to say that he had been a patient of Derek's. Of course, I hadn't been aware of this because a psychotherapist is bound by confidentiality rules. The editor said that the help Derek had given him had changed his life and got him back on track – and that he'd recommended Derek to another family member, who had been heading for a breakdown and said Derek had saved them from that path. I read this message to Derek over the phone while he was in the coma because I wanted him to be aware of the good he'd done. I would say to him, 'These people need you and love you and are all here waiting for you to come back.'

There were friends who'd been coming to see him ever since he was first sick. Ben Wegg-Prosser had supported him and me from the start, visiting him several times in hospital (when he was allowed), as well as at home. Recently our best man, Henry, has seen him too, as has Gloria De Piero, who first introduced us. Another friend, Benjamin Fry, even travelled out to Mexico to sit with Derek when I'd had to return home to take care of the kids. Their love for Derek was never in doubt but sometimes he was only really 'present' for ten minutes at a time and we couldn't predict when those ten minutes might be so it was hard to make arrangements around that. I didn't want anyone to be disappointed when they'd taken the time to come and see him.

If the subject of friends visiting came up, Derek

would say, 'Not yet, not yet.' I understood that he didn't feel ready to see them because he knew he couldn't communicate. There was a sense, too, that he wanted to be at his best when he saw people after such a long time. I felt I would also need to be there to facilitate, because I could act as a translator and make the whole situation more comfortable for everyone. It's a shock for anyone when they first see him after a long time. Whereas I've seen incremental changes over the course of three years, for them it's something of a slap in the face to see how changed he is all at once.

I decided that we had to get through this barrier. Exposing Derek to this felt like a risk – in the same way, it had been a risk for us to go to Mexico and to see Elton John, but at least then I felt I'd been able provide some sort of protective buffer. What I'm realising now is that while I will always be the physical buffer for Derek and be there to care for him, if he is to have any kind of life of his own, he will have to go through some emotional pain – and I can't always spare him that.

When I rang his friends and explained what I was attempting to achieve, every single one leapt at the chance to get involved. It became clear that I had been underestimating the strength of their love for him, which made me feel bad. Before I knew it, a roster was in place with long enough gaps between the visits to ensure that Derek wasn't overwhelmed – and we are adding more and more people to the roster all the time. Even though it's been challenging, I can already see the positive effect it is having on Derek, and how it's opening up the possibility of expanding his world.

Seeing Derek with his friends made me think about how I needed to make time to see my friends too. One thing the kids have observed is that, perhaps understandably, I am noticeably happier when Derek's had a good day – which means that my happiness is dependent on Derek's recovery, which is not fair on anyone. To ensure that we are still entwined and yet have the freedom to flourish in our own ways (as those in any healthy relationship should), I have to work on letting go of the guilt I feel if I spend any time away from him. While I haven't been able to completely do that, I have called up my friends and said, 'I'm ready. I need some fun.' So we are planning some girls' nights out.

Richard Arnold was amazing and told me he was going to bring his party to me. 'We're going to put days in the diary and if Derek is in a good place and wants to be with us, that's great, and if he's not, then we'll just sit in your garden for an hour or go out somewhere local.'

Charlotte Hawkins, Ranvir Singh and I are planning some dates for the autumn and winter and Susanna Reid said, 'Leave it with me, I've got you covered.' We all know these plans might not come to fruition because of Derek's needs but we realise the importance of getting something in the diary, so that there are bright spots on the horizon that are about our friendship. Even if a planned three-hour lunch ends up being half an hour, it's still a conscious decision to do something for us.

If the goal was to let Derek be Derek as he was now, I also had to try not to cling on to things from our life before. I began to declutter the house, to gradually let go of the past, while still holding on to things that are important for Derek and for us now. So, it was time to think about what to do with those worn Birkenstocks by the front door. Seeing them there while he'd been in the coma had been somehow reassuring, as if we were keeping them for him to come back to and slip on. They had gone from being something to treasure, a symbol of hope to something tragic, a reminder of what he still couldn't do. I haven't thrown them away; I've just moved them inside his wardrobe. We are not giving up on the idea of him walking again, but the fact that he can't currently use them doesn't hit me or the kids as soon as we walk in the door any more. I've kept all his Panama hats hanging on the peg in the hall. The Lego Death Star that he and Bill were working on when he got sick is still in Derek's room and they sometimes do little bits of it together, or Derek will watch Bill doing it.

I've recycled all the copies of the *Financial Times* we once collected, in the hope that he would read them when he came home. We still get a *Financial Times* and we read a bit together, or I read bits to him – we try and share it – but I'm letting go and accepting that it's not as it used to be. It was great then but it doesn't work in the same way anymore.

I also had to accept that the pain Derek was in and the stress we were all experiencing weren't going to go away quickly. I couldn't get rid of them entirely, however hard I worked on making him or myself feel better. As time went on, I hoped we could focus less on waiting for things to change, and more on living as well as we could in the circumstances we found ourselves in.

From a medical point of view, we don't know what the future holds. We are currently trying new treatments, which we're hoping will have a positive outcome. We're going back to Mexico to continue his treatment there, and the specialists have every hope that this time we'll see more improvement. Ultimately, we still believe that he can improve and there's no reason not to believe that, but we now know, three years in, that it's not going to be quick, and we are finding ways to exist as a family while the journey continues. Every day it feels like we're making progress on that front.

One day not long ago, we were back in hospital, waiting to find out why his blood tests had come up with some unusual and worrying results. It was very hot, and he had an infection which led to his temperature spiking. He was drifting into sleep and then suddenly jerking awake. Out of the blue, he said to me, 'I wish our Volvo hadn't been stolen. I loved that car.'

'Yeah, I wish it hadn't been stolen, too,' I said. 'We need to find something more accessible, don't we? Something we can transport you in more easily. Maybe we should look at cars together when you're feeling stronger.'

'Yes, I'd like that,' he said. 'I want to look for myself.'

This was positive, I thought.

He closed his eyes and went back to sleep.

Eventually, in the early hours of the morning, Derek was allowed to go home. On the journey back he said, 'I'd like to watch our wedding video again.'

'Really?' I said, surprised, as I thought it might be painful to watch but he urged, 'Yes.'

When we got back, the kids got up, because they were worried about their dad. I told them, 'By the way, kids, Dad would like to watch our wedding video. You two haven't really seen it, have you?'

Darcey had seen it when she was very young, but Billy never had.

I said that perhaps we could watch it the following day but Derek was insistent we watch it that night. They looked at me with slight disbelief and said, 'Okay.'

It was absolutely extraordinary; such a strange feeling to see Derek on that special day.

'Oh my God, Dad, you look so cool!' Darcey and Billy exclaimed, not picking up on the fact that he wasn't in a wheelchair, but on the fact that he wasn't wearing his glasses because he used to wear contact lenses back then;

his hair was longer, too and he didn't have a beard, just a little bit of stubble.

'I think you look so much better without glasses, Dad!' said Billy.

And Derek said, 'Maybe I will wear contact lenses again.'

They were talking about differences in their dad that had nothing to do with the illness. They chatted about my nieces, who were our bridesmaids, being tiny little dots (it was 18 years ago!) and how cute they looked. Then they were looking at Granny and Papa and Grandma and Granddad and Darcey said, 'Granddad literally hasn't changed a bit. It's actually freaky,' and then said, 'Dad, you're lucky; you won't change either.'

They weren't consciously avoiding Derek's changed state; they were accepting the Derek who is here now.

We got to the speeches and I braced myself as I knew it would be difficult for Derek to see himself speaking so eloquently when now the words wouldn't come. I wondered if he would want to pause the film but he insisted on carrying on.

I hadn't remembered every detail of Derek's speech, but of course I knew that it had been phenomenal. We watched as Derek stood up and made his absolutely brilliant, hilarious speech. He took the mickey out of Gloria De Piero, who had introduced us to each other. At one point he said, 'Actually, Kate does the impression of Gloria better – those of you who know Kate well will know that it's very important to script in moments when she wants to interrupt.' (It's true, I always interrupt everybody, all the time!)

So I then did my impression of Gloria when she had said to me, 'I'm having an epiphany – you and Derek Draper!'

He talked about what he saw as this weird TV world I inhabited and the telly talk that bemused him. He watched me on TV and didn't understand why, every two seconds, I would say, 'Still to come ...' and then he realised it was some bit of televisual furniture that indicated that we were going to an ad break ... which made the half of the room not involved in TV really laugh!

Everyone was both moved and in stitches by his words – and watching it again, Derek and the three of us were crying and laughing too.

There were political gags and lots about our family: how both sets of parents had shown us what true love was; how they were still very much in love and supported each other through thick and thin. Derek had said, 'I can't quite believe that Kate agreed to marry me, I'm so lucky, but I'm going to stick with her through thickand thin. As he wound up, he said, 'I'd like to raise a glass to my bride, the new Mrs Draper, and say that I've never felt so happy and so safe, and so cared for in my life.'

At this point, Darcey said, 'Well, she's still doing that, isn't she, Dad?'

Derek looked at me and said, 'I'm sorry.'

I turned to him and said, 'No, I think what you've made clear is what we are doing now is what we've always been about,' I said. 'We've been here to care for each other, through thick and thin.'

At the very end of his wedding speech, Derek said, 'So in the language of Kate's freaky television world, if you think it's been good so far, Kate, let me just say, still to come, still to come …'

The video came to an end and I said to the kids, 'Right, you two, I know there's no school tomorrow, but get to bed.' When they had gone, I turned to Derek and said, 'Right, let's get you to bed too.'

'I want to watch the sun come up,' he said.

I couldn't believe he wanted to stay up – I thought he must be exhausted from having been in hospital and from all the excitement and emotion of the wedding video – but I sensed he needed to. I opened the curtains so he could see the sunrise out of the window.

It gradually got lighter and, as the new day dawned, the sun appeared like a hard orange ball in the sky. As it hoved into view, we were both tearful.

'When is this all going to end?' he said, not really looking at me.

'What do you mean?'

'Everything – the hospital, the pain, all of it,' he said.

'I honestly don't know,' I replied. 'That's what I think I've learned; that I haven't got any answers. But what

I do know is that we will keep trying to get through it together. And we will get there. It will get better. There will come a point.'

'I don't know if I believe that anymore.'

'Well, if you don't believe it, then it won't happen,' I said, squeezing his hand. 'Because I know now that I can't make this happen *for* you – you have to believe it too.'

He carried on looking at the ever-pinkening sky and said, 'Understand.'

There were many things I didn't know the answer to. I didn't know how his health was going to be. I didn't know if I could continue to support him at home physically, myself, or whether our care support would even continue. What I did know was that we were entwined and bound by love. We sat together looking at the sunrise, such an emblem of hope and new beginnings: absolutely together, holding hands; but also apart, thinking about what our own futures held. With the beautiful sunrise glowing outside, he turned to look at me and mouthed, 'Thank you. I love you.' And then, with what I thought was a wry smile, 'Still to come, still to come ...'

Acknowledgements

Sitting down to write a list of everyone I want to thank in helping get *The Strength of Love* to you, I realised it could go on forever – and be longer than the book itself! But special commendations and thanks for getting it over the line, have to start with Michelle Signore and Rebecca Cripps, as well as Madiya Altaf, Eleanor Stammeijer, Natalia Cacciatore and all at Bonnier for their endless patience, nerves of steel and incredible talent when every drama with Derek's health has meant writing has had to stop.

To Matt Nicholls, and the team at United Agents, particularly Tom Kehoe, Zoe Ross and Olivia Davies. To Max Dundas and James Delamare. To Neill Thompson Emma Gormley , Paula Thomas, Katie Rawcliffe, Leanne Clarke, Ceri Aston, Kevin Lygo at ITV. To my Smooth

Radio producer Claire Lynch and James Daniels, Sally Ardis, James Rea. John Chittenden, Ashley Tabor and all at Global Radio.

To my second family at *GMB*: Ben Shephard, Susanna Reid, Richard Arnold, Ranvir Singh, Charlotte Hawkins, Laura Tobin, Sean Fletcher and all behind the scenes who I love to bits and couldn't have done this without.

To my exceptional parents, Gordon and Marylyn Garraway and wonderful brother Matthew. To Dianne and Susan, Ken and Chrina Draper and of course to Derek and to our children, Darcey and Billy, who amaze me every day.